BREASTFEEDING HANDBOOK

BREASTFEEDING HANDBOOK

*A Practical Reference for Physicians, Nurses,
and Other Health Professionals*

JOHANNA GOLDFARB, M.D.

EDITH TIBBETTS

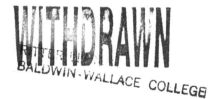
ENSLOW PUBLISHERS

Hillside, New Jersey 07205

The authors thank the following for their help
with the illustrations:

Sue MacGregor
Judy White
Linda Zeimer

Copyright © 1980 by Enslow Publishers, Inc.

All rights reserved.

Library of Congress Cataloging in Publication Data

Goldfarb, Johanna.
  Breastfeeding Handbook.

  Bibliography: p.
  Includes index.
  1. Breast feeding. I. Tibbetts, Edith, joint author.
II. Title. [DNLM: 1. Breast feeding—Handbooks.
WS125 M911b]

RJ216.G64   649'.3   79-20601

ISBN 0-89490-030-7

Printed in the United States of America

10 9 8 7 6 5 4 3 2 1

CONTENTS

FOREWORD

by
Lewis A. Barness, M.D.

Professor and Chairman
Department of Pediatrics
College of Medicine
University of South Florida
Tampa, Florida

Combining a sensitive approach to the nursing mother and infant with factual information on the physiology of nursing, the nutritional value of human milk, and short answers to problems which may arise, the authors have produced a text that is useful to all who care for infants and pregnant women.

After many years of artificially feeding infants, an important number of infants is being breastfed. During the interval of little nursing, parents as well as doctors, nurses and other caretakers forgot many of the tricks as well as the travails of successful nurturing. A comprehensive text became necessary because, although "breast is best" and "cow's milk is for the calf," nursing mothers may develop problems—and breastfeeding infants require observation and examination periodically to be certain that the feeding regimen is suitable for that infant and his parents.

Just as the movement away from nursing to artificial feeding was fostered by non-professionals, so also the return to nursing has been fostered by groups of lay women. While their interest may have been largely encouraged by a wish to return to nature, considerable evidence has developed to indicate the superiority of breastfeeding nutritionally and immunologically. As the authors point out, there also may be some psychological advantage to nursing. Nonetheless, the authors are careful to note that regardless of the type of feeding selected, the adviser can best serve the welfare of parents and child by encouraging the parents to decide on their desired feeding regimen after objective descriptions of advantages and disadvantages of varied feeding regimens—and then supporting the decision.

Whereas it may be that good artificial formulas are still less expensive to make than the cost of nursing, with ever rising energy demands we may soon see an almost universal return to nursing. Leisurely reading of this volume and later going back to it as a reference may obviate many anticipated difficulties and give the professional the needed confidence to advise for successful nurturing.

Lewis A. Barness

*   *   *

FOREWORD

by
Ronald A. Chez, M.D.

Professor and Chairman
Department of Obstetrics and Gynecology
Milton S. Hershey Medical Center
The Pennsylvania State University

Looking back to my early days as an obstetrician-gynecologist, the over-riding attitude about the care of the newborn was that "time zero" was the moment of delivery. The major decisions were made at that moment: whether to circumcise, what to name the baby, whether to breastfeed, and more. The mother frequently had to decide on the delivery room table whether to breastfeed or not, so that the appropriate medications could be administered. I recall this with no sense of inferiority, because those of us who practiced then were as dedicated, honest, committed, and confident in our knowledge as those who practice today. Probably those who start 10 years from now will look back upon those in the forefront of today's medicine and regard us as having had quaint and not very profound thoughts—and little understanding of "natural processes."

Breastfeeding Handbook makes the point nicely that care of the newborn should start in early pregnancy or even before conception. With regard to breastfeeding, there are important ways that the mother can prepare herself before delivery. All of us should recognize and remember that the present goal of a 24-28 lb weight gain during pregnancy is designed for the laying down of appropriate fat reserves for the subsequent caloric requirements of the production of breast milk.

The woman who actively participates in her own care, who makes an effort to establish a dialogue with her health-care professional, and who takes the initiative to learn about the normal and abnormal processes going on in her body will be able to extract the very best from the already very good health-care system. The challenge to health-care professionals is to be current, informed, knowledgeable and communicative.

This book has a number of pearls that are not easily found elsewhere. It supplies the answers to clinical problems, which serve as a basis for one's own collection of anecdotal data. All the answers are not here—nor should they be. The few that aren't should be supplied through the tenet of individualized patient care.

Ronald A. Chez

* * *

FOREWORD

by
Reginald Lightwood, M.D., F.R.C.P., D.P.H.

Consulting Physician to the Hospital for
Sick Children, Great Ormond Street
and
Consulting Paediatrician to St. Mary's Hospital
University of London
England

Good nutrition throughout the life of a child is fundamental to his health. And yet, surprisingly enough, recent generations of paediatricians in the Western countries, although they usually have excellent knowledge of disease and of many rare syndromes, show scant interest in the principles of nutrition, and are little able to explain to mothers and nursing personnel the physiological advantages of breastfeeding over bottle feeding.

In England and Wales a publication in 1978 by the Department of Health showed that 25 per cent of mothers had heard no mention of breastfeeding. Surely, the obstetrician should instruct the mother-to-be in the preparation of her breasts and nipples, and the paediatrician should see her soon after the birth of the baby in order to discuss the management of breastfeeding.

Fortunately, there is now in the Western countries evidence of a resurgence of interest in breastfeeding and a recent increase in knowledge of the nutritional and immunological superiority of breast milk. In the developing countries breastfeeding is almost universal in the rural areas, but many of the people have moved into the urban areas in search of work, where artificial feeding has increased in imitation of the habits of Western countries and as a result of the promotion of sales of artificial foods by commerce.

In consequence, there has been an alarming increase in the incidence of gastroenteritis in the cities of the developing countries.

Lack of teaching in regard to nutrition is a weakness of the curriculum in most medical schools in the United Kingdom as in the United States. When the doctors meet classes of student midwives and nurses they usually open with the statement that breastfeeding is best, and the rest of the lecture is devoted to the mechanics of bottle feeding. The explanation is that most of these medical teachers have not had the benefit of experience of breastfeeding and the medical schools have given them insufficient teaching about the physiology of nutrition and breastfeeding.

The advantages of breast milk are many, especially its immunological value in protecting the infant from infection.

11

A class of pupil midwives and nurses should be given three or four times as much teaching time on breastfeeding as on the techniques of artificial feeding. They should be taught about the gradual introduction of mixed feeding at about four to five months of age. They should be taught about infantile obesity.

The information in this book will be a good basis for teaching what is true and what is false in infant feeding.

Reginald Lightwood

*   *   *

A NOTE TO THE READER

Increasing numbers of Western women and babies are finding the special joys that come with successful breastfeeding. But reports of women giving up breastfeeding within the first month, and reports of babies who fail to thrive on breast milk, are disturbing. While we are seeing more and more articles in the medical literature that convince us that "breast is best," practical information on breastfeeding management techniques that could help more women to nurse successfully is not available. For this reason, we have compiled such information and written this handbook. It is our purpose to present a concise, complete reference for practicing pediatricians, obstetricians, family practitioners, registered nurses, nurse practitioners, medical students, breastfeeding counselors and other health professionals who care for the "nursing couple," that is, the nursing mother and her infant. Perhaps not all who choose to breastfeed will succeed, but it is our belief that no woman should fail for lack of sound advice and encouragement.

We hope we have supplied the needed information; the support and encouragement must be added.

We wish to emphasize that this handbook is not a description of what the breastfeeding experience is like typically. In order to give solutions to breastfeeding problems, most that can occur—even those that occur only rarely—are described. We hope that this description of problems will not dissuade any reader from wanting to experience the joys of breastfeeding. Many of the problems described in this handbook are unlikely to occur when the right information and support are given.

We see this handbook as a reference tool with different sections, to which the professional can turn quickly for information. We felt that the handbook would be most useful to the reader if each chapter contained the needed information on that subject. Thus at times we have repeated information in more than one chapter, so that it could be most easily located.

The Handbook has two parts: the first section, including a chapter on the pharmacology of drugs in breast milk by Dr. Cheston Berlin, contains background information that can help the reader to understand breastfeeding. We have chosen to keep this first section brief. The second and larger section, the heart of the handbook, is on management. There we have included information on managing the normal course of lactation and also information on managing the problems that are alluded to above. We have tried to present practical information, including some that has not previously been widely circulated in the medical literature.

Perhaps the best way to use this handbook is to use the facts presented along with the notion that successful breastfeeding happens when it is consciously nurtured.

We begin this book by stressing the role of education for newly breastfeeding women. Various immediate causes for lactation failure have been noted (failure to condition the let-down reflex, inadequate milk supply with resulting failure to thrive in the infant, painful engorgement, soreness, mastitis, etc.) A serious and broader study of human lactation (success and failure) requires one to look further. *Why* do Western women not have enough milk, fail to condition their let-down reflex, or develop painful breast problems? In almost all cases of lactation failure, the women do not have a source of basic information and emotional support (1,2). They do not understand the mechanism of breastfeeding. It is this lack of information (together with lack of support) we suggest that is the overriding and pre-eminent cause of failure.

		low milk supply		
		or	*which*	
lack of information	*leads to* →	poor let-down	*in turn* →	lactation
and support		or	*lead to*	failure
		breast problems		

Women with support and information may develop problems, but rarely problems so severe that lactation fails.

Instead of focusing primarily on specific cures for let-down or other problems, one must focus on giving generalized information and support. Although we do list specific solutions in this handbook, we urge that such specifics be used within a framework of giving generalized support to the woman. Unless we do so, today's specific problem is likely to be followed by another different problem tomorrow.

As the British physician Mavis Gunther has said, "One teaches the mother to understand lactation." (3) The mother who has been so taught, who does understand a few, very simple principles, such as how to maintain an adequate milk supply by nursing frequently is likely to nurse successfully throughout the early weeks. On the other hand, the woman whose instruction in breastfeeding is limited only to specific information, such as advice on nipple care or advice on how many minutes per breast each early nursing should last, is less likely to continue nursing successfuly. Such an uninstructed mother lacks a basic understanding of lactation and is in a weak position to manage her own breastfeeding situation at home with the baby. While giving the mother a cure for sore nipples (or telling her how many minutes to nurse) helps her to get through today, teaching her to understand lactation helps her to breastfeed for weeks or months.

We hope to show that this helpful teaching is neither difficult nor time-consuming, nor does it involve technical information. It can be as simple as saying, "When the baby doesn't seem satisfied, nurse more frequently for a couple of days to build up your milk supply."

We do not attempt to dictate the best course of lactation. We feel that most decisions concerning child care, including those about the course of lactation, are best made by informed parents. We see the health professional ideally as a well-informed source of information, alternatives and support. Questions such as whether the baby ought to be accustomed to an occasional bottle, when it is best to wean a child, or how parents should respond to night awakenings are decisions parents should make in view of their own particular family needs. We can provide specific information about the ease or difficulty of weaning at various ages but we feel the mother must decide for herself whether the rewards and problems of prolonged nursing are worthwhile.

There is, however, one issue on which we cannot remain neutral—that is, the need for frequent nursings, especially in early lactation. We too have heard and read that nursing frequently, on demand, is impractical and too tiring for the modern Western woman with many other responsibilities and needs. But what else can one do with a crying infant that is so easy (and so beneficial to conditioning the let-down reflex and to building the milk supply) as to sit or lie down to nurse? The common alternatives such as rocking the baby, pushing a baby carriage, offering a pacifier or bottle, or listening to the baby's cries are certainly not so easy as nursing.

Although we recognize the importance of a supportive husband and father and have included the father in some sections, we have tried to avoid making the traditional assumption that all breastfeeding women are married. Increasingly they are not.

We add what has become a common apology for referring to all babies as "he" or "him," while the mother is "she" and "her." This is merely to simplify the usage of pronouns.

We spell breastfeeding as one word, bottle feeding as two and give credit for this distinction to Dr. Dana Raphael: "Breastfeeding is a physiological fact, like heartbeat; bottle feeding is a method, like spoon feeding (4)."

References

1. Ladas, A: How to help mothers breastfeed, Clin. Ped. 9:12, 1970.

2. Raphael, D: *The Tender Gift: Breastfeeding.* Englewood Cliffs, NJ: Prentice Hall, 1973.

3. Gunther, M: The New Mother's View of Herself. CIBA Foundation Symposium no. 45: 145, 1976.

4. Raphael, D, ed., The Lactation Review II (1), 1977.

Chapter 1

An Overview of Breastfeeding

RECENT TRENDS IN WESTERN COUNTRIES

While there was a movement away from breastfeeding in the Western World earlier this century, in recent years the trend has been reversed. Surveys show that increasing numbers of women are choosing to breastfeed. A recent survey (1977) in the United States indicated that about one-half of newborns discharged from maternity hospitals are being at least partially breastfed (1) compared to estimates for earlier years of 18% in 1966, 21% in 1956, and 38% in 1946 (2).

Lactation Failure

If one inquires about the degree of success in *maintaining* lactation beyond the neonatal period, however, the figures are not so positive. A young woman trying to breastfeed her newborn infant today stands a fair chance of experiencing lactation failure, especially if she believes that the breastfeeding process will continue "naturally."

Many women who choose to breastfeed stop nursing within a few days or weeks. Studies on the prevalence of breastfeeding in the Western countries suggest that often it is of only a token nature, that breastfeeding is combined with the use of bottles, or that it is concluded prematurely. In two British surveys, of the women who were breastfeeding at the time of discharge from the hospital, only 50% were still breastfeeding at two months postpartum (3,4).

Even more striking, a survey in London showed that 50% of mothers who were breastfeeding at the time of discharge from the hospital weaned by three weeks, some failing during the first week (5).

In another survey, "well informed" (about breastfeeding) British women were found more likely to continue nursing than "uninformed" women. The most common reason for stopping breastfeeding was a belief by the mother that she had "insufficient milk." (6) Similarly, in a small survey of mothers who gave up breastfeeding prematurely in South Wales, the most common explanation was a belief by the mothers that they were producing insufficient milk (7).

Lactation failure in Ireland, which was defined as a rapid decline in the breastfeeding rate during the early weeks at home, was believed to be related to a lack of maternal support (8).

Breastfeeding success or failure in Australia was found to be related to the type of care and the degree of understanding given to new mothers by medical attendants, with many women failing (9).

Although Sweden has traditionally had a high rate of breastfeeding, a decline also has been reported there. In 1944, 56% of Swedish infants were being breastfed at the age of six months, while in 1970 only 7% were, according to official statistics. In one study on the duration of breastfeeding in the first 24 weeks postpartum, the percentage of women breastfeeding dropped from 89.6% to 4%. Many women in this study breastfed briefly despite a clear wish to continue longer; the most common reason for terminating breastfeeding was a belief that the "milk dried up." (10)

Similarly, women in the United States who initiate breastfeeding may continue to do so only briefly. In a study of "highly select" women who had higher than average levels of education and income and who were attending prenatal classes at suburban Boston hospitals, 42% were unable to overcome problems. The three most common reasons for early weaning were "not enough milk," "I always felt tired," and "Baby's doctor told me to stop." (11)

This syndrome of early lactation failure in modern society is a painful one, as can perhaps be demonstrated by the personal record that follows:

> Like magic it happened. With a surge, three days after the birth of my first child, my breasts became distended with milk. I had naively assumed throughout my pregnancy that when the infant arrived I would automatically be ready to feed him, and that it was as simple as that. But my joy turned to anguish as the baby screamed angrily when there was not enough milk. Little did I know that I had begun the terrifying cycle so familiar to many mothers who had tried for the first time to breastfeed.
>
> When the baby was but a week old, I became really anxious. The baby cried louder. I strained to feed. The baby got nothing, and I got more frightened. Finally, screaming with frustration, the baby turned away. Panic-stricken, I did the one thing I had promised myself I would never do. I prepared a bottle.

> The "magic" of breastfeeding? As far as I was concerned it was more like sorcery, for without warning, a short time later my milk disappeared altogether (12).

The Committee on Nutrition of the American Academy of Pediatrics and the Nutrition Committee of the Canadian Paediatric Society recommend that, ideally, breast milk should be practically the only source of nutrients for the first four to six months (13). This is certainly not met when breastfeeding stops prematurely.

Why are women failing? Are Western women really producing too little milk? Why do women in less complex societies continue to breastfeed successfully? Lactation failure is not unknown in those societies: there, too, women have breastfeeding problems—but the problems generally are solved.

BRIEF HISTORY OF INFANT FEEDING (16,17)

In considering the causes of lactation failure in modern times, it may be useful to review the history of infant feeding. It has been postulated that there is a correlation between eras during which women are objects of amusement (rather than real contributors to the work of the societies) and eras during which large numbers of upper class women reject breastfeeding by using wet nurses or artificial feeds (13). Throughout history there have been many eras during which women have sought an alternate method of infant nutrition. While in Hebraic tradition only the child of a mother who had died or who could not nurse her own was given to a wet nurse, in ancient Greece and Rome the wealthy routinely had their infants wet-nursed, most often by well-cared-for and respected slaves. The use of animal milk as well began at this same time but was much less common. Egyptian and Indian writings describe the attributes of a good wet nurse, as well as tests for purity of human milk.

The lack of concern for children which characterized early industrialization in Europe reached its worst in the 17th and 18th centuries. For the first time working people as well as the rich turned away from breastfeeding. They used artificial feeds in the form of paps (broths of grains and water) and panadas (broths made of combinations of flour, grain, water, butter and, occasionally, animal milk.) Women forced to work to survive saw no alternative. Children often were abandoned or poorly cared for. Infant mortality soared.

Prior to the 1900's, the use of cows' milk was associated with high risk of death from diarrheal disease, undoubtedly partly because of bacterial contamination.

The 1800's saw improved conditions for children in Europe and a renewed trend back to breastfeeding. The wealthy still had the option of using a wet nurse, but this was increasingly less popular. Infant mortality fell.

Pediatrics became a separate specialty, and with this there was increasing interest in the diseases and welfare of children. Research in the early 1900's into infant nutrition resulted in the production of cows' milk that was usable in making safe infant formulas. Many felt these formulas to be the equivalent of breast milk.

Ever-improving technology has allowed private industry to continue to develop multiple, safe, standardized infant formulas so that today many varieties exist throughout Europe and America. This new availability of what appeared to be a safe alternative to breastmilk, combined with increased interest in the rights of women, after World War I began a trend away from breastfeeding. Pediatric texts turned from descriptions of the normal course of lactation to descriptions of infant formulas and associated health complications (which became increasingly common).

Obstetrical practices were changing also. Increasingly babies in the 20th century West were born in hospitals, often with the mother fully anaesthetized. It was not unusual for a mother to first see her newborn 24 hours after the actual delivery. Father waited patiently alone in the modern hospital and viewed his sterilely wrapped infant through the glass window of a modern centralized nursery. Babies were sleepy from anaesthesia and were fed (after a prolonged fast) by nurses. Nurses' schedules made infant-feeding schedules a necessity. Babies were found to tolerate four hours between formula feeds well.

The bottle in the 20th century became a symbol of woman's freedom and of the "modern" way. Sterilizing bottles, measuring milk, corn syrup and water, and juggling the formula composition was judged easier than breastfeeding. It did mean that someone other than the mother could feed the baby, and that as a consequence she could go out alone and could therefore more easily work outside the home. This was an era of strict child discipline. Rocking chairs and cradles were frowned upon as habit forming. Babies, it was believed, should be fed on rigid schedules, and letting the baby cry was better than spoiling him with frequent feedings and cuddling.

As the population became more mobile, the nuclear family evolved, with the young couple living away from extended family support. The trend of women leaving the home has continued to the present day. Maternity leaves often were and still are usually brief, women priding themselves on how quickly they can get back to work after the birth of a child. The worth of a woman increasingly today appears to be determined by her role outside of her home; it is in her profession. Many women must work for economic reasons alone, however. Simultaneously, the increased numbers of "ready to feed" formulas and improved packaging have made formula preparation easier and safer.

That breastfeeding is a comfort to the child and a pleasurable experience to the mother was forgotten during the mid 20th century. Somehow, breastfeeding and bottle feeding became accepted as equivalents. Breastfeeding as a normal sexual function of women became largely ignored and seemed to have lost its image of beauty. Breastfeeding as a loving bond between two human beings was largely forgotten in a culture where women's breasts were to be hidden, as sexual objects for the pleasure of husbands and lovers only. The woman who modestly nursed her infant often was considered embarrassing, even animalistic. She had to be hidden in the bedroom or ladies' room, while the woman who dressed provocatively to reveal most of her breasts was socially acceptable.

Increasingly, during the mid 20th century, those few women who, despite negative influences, chose to breastfeed their infants, met with frequent failure. The art of successful breastfeeding seemed to have been largely lost.

In the Third World

Infant feeding practices revolving around bottle feeding had become generally accepted as the modern way in Western countries. The next step was exporting. Along with the other so-called advantages of Western technology, powdered formula and the feeding bottle were exported—and accepted by some native populations along with other symbols of the modern world. Large corporations saw the Third World as a new market in which they could profitably sell powdered formula. In some cases, native women dressed in white uniforms actively sought to promote formula and bottle feeding to new mothers.

Although the native women began to believe that the bottle would be as good for their babies as it was for Western babies, they often could not afford to buy adequate amounts of the powdered formula to put into the bottle. In underdeveloped countries, a considerable percentage of the family's income might be required to feed the youngest and least productive member. Feeding one four-month old infant in Guatemala would require almost 80% of the per capita income (18). The usual solution is for the mother to overdilute the formula; in some cases, a four-day supply is stretched to last from five days to three weeks (18).

There are further problems. Families in Third World countries generally have no source of uncontaminated water to use in formula preparation, no refrigeration and no knowledge of proper formula preparation. Their bottle-fed babies are at high risk for malnutrition, infection and death. The large multi-national corporations that profited from the sale of formula were criticized.

The issue continues to be a heated emotional one. Yet the entire blame for the infant malnutrition, mortality and morbidity cannot be ascribed to the corporations, nor to the bottle. The malnourished women of many Third World countries can fully support the growth of their infants with breast milk for 3 to 4 months at most. Ideally, the mother needs to be fed well so that she can nurse optimally, but nutritious and relatively inexpensive weaning foods and supplemental formula may also have an appropriate role. In some cases the welfare of the entire family depends on the mother's returning to work. The baby must then be left in the care of a grandmother or an older child, and again, supplemental foods may be necessary. Blaming the bottle feeding alone is an oversimplification of the complex issue of malnutrition:

> The effects of poverty—lack of food and safe drinking water,
> the absence of sanitation and health care, political indiffer-
> ence to mothers in poverty—are the determinants of diseases
> and death of infants in the developing world (19).

In some developing countries, government policies increasingly promote breastfeeding, and the regulation of the promotion and sale of formulas, in an attempt to decrease infant mortality and morbidity.

WHY THE RETURN TO BREASTFEEDING IN WESTERN COUNTRIES?

The past decade in Western culture has seen a renewed interest in all things natural. Increasingly the present generation of young people feels that nature's way is often best. This change of attitude coincides with an increasing interest in natural childbirth principles and in the importance of mother-infant interactions for child development. There also has been a trend away from rigid schedules and strict discipline for the infant. (These trends do not negate the importance of scientific research. The "noble savage" does not always know best: the use of analgesia/anaesthesia during labor and delivery often is appropriate, and a newborn can thrive on infant formula.)

Scientific investigation is demonstrating that bottle feeding does not equal breastfeeding. They are equivalent neither nutritionally nor immunologically. Babies have thrived on formula for several generations and will continue to do so, but many lay people and professionals are beginning to understand that breastfeeding is optimal for the normal mother and baby.

The return to breastfeeding in the past decade has begun as a middle class phenomenon. "Breast is best" sentiment among middle class women sometimes runs so high that even women who find breastfeeding unappealing now feel pressured by their peers to nurse their babies (although briefly). Larger numbers of breastfeeding women have brought larger numbers of breastfeeding problems to the physician's attention.

WHAT MEASURES HAVE BEEN EFFECTIVE IN FOSTERING BREASTFEEDING?

Although Western culture in the mid 20th century has not been particularly effective in supporting breastfeeding for the recommended minimum of four to six months, there have been some notable exceptions. In order to gain insight for improving the outcome in the future, it seems appropriate to ask how and why these exceptions have been successful.

The Doula

In our culture we say a baby is born; the child's birth shifts our interest away from mother to baby. In many cultures, it is said that at parturition, a woman becomes a mother, keeping the emphasis on the mother. Dana Raphael, an anthropologist, has noted that in these cultures where breastfeeding is common and successful, there is a special system of support for the new mother. It is recognized that a young woman *learns* to mother. She learns how to care for her new baby; it is not an assumed ability. In societies where mother's milk is the only available safe source of infant nutrition, the child's life depends on his mother's ability to nurse. In every culture studied by Dr. Raphael, a person or persons, usually female, often the woman's mother, is assigned the care of a new mother. Her job is to "mother the mother." She takes over household chores, cares for the woman and, most important, supports the young mother as she learns to nurse her new infant. Dr. Raphael has called this person the "doula" (12) or helper. Western culture lacks this concept of "matrescence" (becoming-a-mother) and provides no doula.

Modern women often are alone in the first, vital days and weeks of lactation. Grandma, if she is there, may never have nursed a baby. It is during this crucial period that women need emotional support and correct information on technique if they are to learn the pleasures of a nursing relationship and to avoid the anguish of lactation failure.

Dr. Raphael has suggested a solution for Western women—reciprocal doulas (12). Two pregnant women who are due several months from each other make arrangements to serve as doulas to each other.

Some women have found that a book on breastfeeding, especially the book *Nursing Your Baby* by Karen Pryor, is a source of information and support; the book appears partially to fill the role of the doula.

Lay Groups

Some women have found the support and information needed to succeed at breastfeeding in lay support groups. La Leche League International (LLLI) is the largest and best known of the breastfeeding support groups, although there are others. Joining La Leche League has helped many women and their babies to enjoy a successful breastfeeding experience (20).

Support groups supply information about breastfeeding in terms that mothers can understand. The importance of someone to call on for advice and encouragement about breastfeeding is greatest in the first weeks, but continues throughout the course of lactation. Although many women are affiliated with a group, many more are not. Some women do not like to obtain information through group membership, or are unable to locate one nearby.

Supportive Physicians

A few physicians have written about how they have helped nursing mothers and babies successfully (21,22,23). They have sometimes credited their knowledge of breastfeeding to their wives or to the nursing mothers in their practices. For physicians as well as lay counselors and doulas, it appears that expertise about breastfeeding techniques most often has come from actual experience. The majority of physicians, however, were not trained in techniques that would have enabled them to help breastfeeding women with practical matters.

Programs Established by Medical Facilities

Some medical facilities have established programs to foster breastfeeding. One medical facility created a program with the following components:

1.   Consistent in-hospital counseling by one professional, a pediatric nurse-practitioner.

2.   Post-discharge telephone contact with the same professional.

3.   A "breastfeeding clinic" for new mothers and their babies conducted by the same practitioner, two weeks after hospital discharge (24).

Summary

In all of the above, emotional support of the new mother and the supplying of information about breastfeeding techniques are common factors leading to success. The mother needs to be given support during the early weeks of lactation. The nurturing of successful breastfeeding must be given a high priority, made a goal that is consciously worked toward. The combination of support plus information has proved more effective than either alone (25).

Personal, first-hand experience with breastfeeding often has played a vital role in training both lay persons and professionals; it will undoubtedly continue to be very important. First-hand experience has been largely the only option for learning some aspects of breastfeeding; medical and nursing schools have not even tried to teach the practical management of breastfeeding. But to believe that first-hand or family experience with breastfeeding is an absolute prerequisite for understanding it is to negate the potential of education. Practical breastfeeding information can be taught. Although personal experience will always be a good source of knowledge, it is not the only option.

For health professionals in complex Western society, there does not seem to be one simple way to encourage breastfeeding, but several effective ones. The following are directed to the health professional as possible suggestions for encouraging breastfeeding.

. . . . .Possible Measures for Encouraging Breastfeeding . . . . .

1. Support a change in public attitude through education in schools and through the media. The importance of education is shown by the fact that women feel they come to a decision about breastfeeding from the personal convictions of themselves and their husbands rather than because of advice from a professional person or acquaintance.

2. Improve education about breastfeeding techniques in medical and nursing schools and in residency training programs of obstetricians, pediatricians, and family practitioners.

3. Physicians and midwives should communicate the advantages of breastfeeding to expectant parents during prenatal care and in classes in prepared childbirth. Practical information should be given as well.

4. Improve the hospital experience.

(a) When possible, decrease sedation in labor and delivery to prevent impaired suckling in the infant during the first days of life.

(b) Avoid separating the mother and infant during the first 24 hours. Encourage early first feedings at the breast.

(c) Encourage rooming-in for all breastfeeding mothers except where special problems exist. Frequent feeds should be ordered for mothers who are unable to have rooming-in, when possible.

(d) Eliminate routine supplemental formula feeds.

(e) Emphasize basic breastfeeding information (such as how to ensure an adequate milk supply) over peripheral advice (such as about bras, creams, fluid intake).

(f) Conduct in-service programs for hospital personnel who work with breastfeeding mothers, to ensure that correct, consistent and basic information is given to new mothers.

(g) Eliminate written materials and free samples given by formula manufacturers. Substitute written materials that contain information on breastfeeding techniques and help to convey to new mothers a basic understanding of breastfeeding.

(h) Consider holding informal classes for new mothers on the postpartum unit to discuss getting started at breastfeeding and to prepare new mothers for the early days at home. Mothers who have nursed previous children successfully can be included and asked "What are some of the things you learned by experience about breastfeeding that you wish someone had told you?" (26)

5.   Schedule the check-up of the newborn after discharge at two weeks postpartum. This can help guarantee early discovery of nursing problems. The visit can provide an opportunity for the new mother to discuss questions and concerns and for the professional to give valuable reassurance and confidence to the mother.

6.   If the first check-up is to be delayed, make arrangements for contacting new mothers by telephone at the beginning of the second week postpartum to detect any early nursing problems. New mothers should be reassured that their telephone calls and questions are truly welcome.

7.   Health professionals should be aware of lay breastfeeding groups in their area. In some cases, new groups are formed, either as a new chapter of an existing group, such as La

Leche, or as a completely new group associated with a medical facility, a childbirth group, or a women's group. Some groups offer only breastfeeding help, others are more general postpartum support groups.

8. Health professionals may want to support efforts to promote maternity leaves of six months duration and nursing breaks during the day.

References

1. Total Breast Milk Shares, Survey based on 1971-1977, Ross Laboratories.

2. Meyer, HF: Breast feeding in the United States, Clin. Pediatr. 7:708, 1968.

3. Sloper, K et al: Factors influencing breast feeding, Arch. Dis. Child. 50:165, 1975.

4. Coles, EC et al: (Letter) Encouraging breast feeding, Lancet. 2:978, 1975.

5. Bax, MCO and Hart, H: (Letter) Encouraging breastfeeding, Lancet. 2:1214, 1975.

6. Eastham, E et al: Further decline of breastfeeding, Br. Med. J. 1:305, 1976.

7. Davies, DP and Thomas, C: Why do women stop breastfeeding? Lancet. 1:420, 1976.

8. Fitzpatrick, C and Kevany, J: The duration of breast feeding, J. Irish Med. Asso. 70:1, 1977.

9. Mobbs, EJ and Mobbs, GA: Breast feeding—success (or failure) due to attendants and not to prevailing fashion, Medical J. of Australia 1:770, 1972.

10. Sjolin, S et al: Factors related to early termination of breast feeding, Acta Paediatr. Scand. 66:505, 1977.

11. Cole, JP: Breastfeeding in the Boston suburbs in relation to personal-social factors, Clin. Pediatr. 16:352, 1977.

12. Raphael, D: *The Tender Gift: Breastfeeding.* Englewood Cliffs, New Jersey: Prentice Hall, 1973.

13. Newton, M and Newton, N: Medical progress: psychologic aspects of lactation, N. Engl. J. Med. 277:1179, 1967.

14. Francis, B: Successful lactation and women's sexuality, J. Trop. Pediatr. 22:4, 1976.

15. American Academy of Pediatrics Committee on Nutrition, Pediatr. 62:591, 1978.

16. Davidson, WD: A brief history of infant feeding, J. Pediatr. 43:74, 1953.

17. Wickes, IG: A history of infant feeding, Arch. Dis. Child. 28:151, 232, 332, 416, 495, 1953.

18. Lappé, FM and Collins, J: *Food First.* Boston: Houghton Mifflin Company, 1977, pp. 312-319.

19. Raphael, D, ed., *The Lactation Review* III (1), 1978.

20. Meara, H: A key to successful breastfeeding in a non-supportive culture, J. Nurse-Midwifery 21 (1), Spring, 1976.

21. Applebaum, RM: The physician and a common sense approach to breast feeding, South Med. J. 63:793, 1970.

22. Kimball, ER: Breast feeding in private practice, Quart. Northwest Univ. Med School 25.257, 1951

23. Kemberling, SR: Supporting breast-feeding, Pediatr. 63:60, 1979.

24. Selby, M: Fostering breastfeeding: a pediatric program, Keeping Abreast Journal II (3), 1977.

25. Ladas, A: How to help mothers breastfeed, Clin. Pediatr. 9 (12), 1970.

26. Bird, IS: Breast-feeding classes on the postpartum unit, Am. J. Nurs. 75:456, 1975.

Chapter 2

Anatomy, Physiology, and Composition of Human Milk

ANATOMY

Maturation of the female breast occurs during puberty, initially under the control of estrogen, and later, when ovulation becomes regular, estrogen and progesterone together. Estrogen is believed to be responsible for the proliferation of epithelial elements (ducts); glandular proliferation requires the combination of estrogen and progesterone (2).

At maturity, the adult female breast consists of about 20 lobes or segments, each connected centrally by a duct to a lactiferous or milk sinus. The sinuses are dilations of the duct system, located in the areola mammae. The ducts connect to nipple pores, which are visible openings on the nipple tip. Each lobe is itself composed of 20 to 40 smaller divisions or lobuli, and each lobule in turn consists of smaller units called alveoli. There are 10 to 100 alveoli per lobule (see Fig. 2-1). The alveoli are the most distal epithelial structures and are the site of proliferation and differentiation of cells into functioning glandular tissue (milk sacs) during pregnancy and lactation. The alveoli and small milk ducts are surrounded or ensheathed by myoepithelial cells (M-E cells). These are cells of ectodermal origin, whose star-shaped branches encircle the alveoli and small ducts. They contain myfibrils which contract under hormonal stimulation of oxytocin, resulting in the reflex "letting-down" stimulation of milk (see the discussion of the let-down reflex later in this chapter). There is sympathetic, but no parasympathetic, innervation of the myoepithelial cells. Sympathetic stimulation causes relaxation of the cells, which results in inhibition of the let-down reflex (see Fig. 2-2).

The lobes or segments of the mature breast are arranged around the

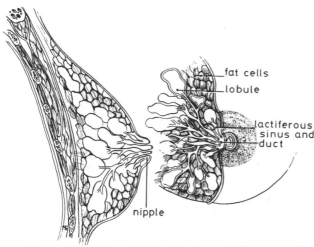

Figure 2-1. Internal anatomy of the breast.

areola and nipple and give the breast its mounded shape. They are supported by connective and fatty tissue and rich vascular and lymphatic networks. The actual size of the breast is related more to the amount of fat present than to the amount of glandular element.

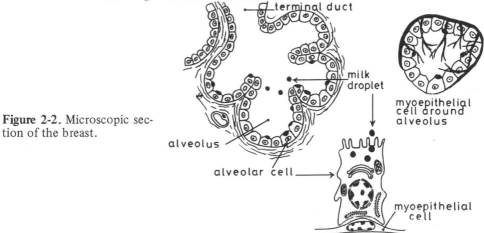

Figure 2-2. Microscopic section of the breast.

Nervous innervation of the breast consists of afferent somatic fibers (which begin in the nipple and areola mammae and which travel via the spinothalamic tracts to the hypothalamus and pituitary) and efferent, or motor fibers, from the sympathetic nervous system (which originate from the thoracic paravertebral sympathetic ganglia). There is no parasympathetic innervation or voluntary motor innervation of the breast.

The rich innervation of the nipple and areola is responsible for the reflex erection of the nipple during tactile or sucking stimulation. The nipple and areola contain smooth muscle cells arranged in rings and also longitudinal strands that contract the areola skin in response to sympathetic nerve stimulation. This results in the nipple becoming erect. Sympathetic fibers also are responsible for reflex vasoconstriction of the arterial blood supply to the breast and, as mentioned, for relaxation of the M-E cells. Opening into the areola are large sebaceous glands (Montgomery glands) and small sebaceous glands. Both secrete substances that lubricate the areola. The Montgomery glands, which are modified mammary glands, proliferate with the hormonal stimulation of puberty and pregnancy and atrophy at menopause (see Fig. 2-3).

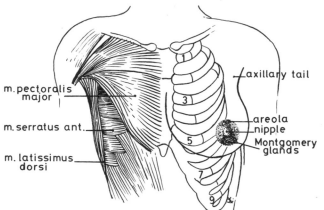

Figure 2-3. Surface anatomy of the breast.

Throughout adult life, ending with menopause, the female breast responds   to the cyclical variation in hormonal levels. Prior to menstruation, under the influence of rising estrogen and progesterone levels, there is limited proliferation of ductular and glandular elements, as well as increased water retention and a mononuclear infiltration of the stroma. With menstruation, hormonal levels fall and there is a diuresis and regression of the cellular changes. With each cycle there is some limited increase in peripheral ductular structure throughout early adulthood.

During pregnancy high levels of estrogen, progesterone, and prolactin, as well as placental-lactogenic hormones, cause further rapid development of the breasts into functioning glandular organs. Increase in breast size (often noted as a sense of fullness or tenderness), visibly dilated superficial veins over the chest, and a darkening and enlarging of the areola, are good clinical signs of pregnancy and reflect hormonal stimulation.   It is estimated that that there is an increase in weight of ¾ to 1½ lb per breast during pregnancy.   Early increases in weight and size reflect increased vascularity (blood supply doubling by the end of pregnancy) and proliferation of distal duct structure. During mid- and late pregnancy, differentiation of the alveolar epithelial cells occurs, with the cells enlarging and becoming metabolically active. Myoepithelial cells also proliferate and encircle the proliferating terminal milk sacs (alveoli) and small ducts. Colostrum is produced from the middle of gestation and accounts for some of the increase in breast size during the second half of pregnancy. If a pregnancy is terminated after the first half of gestation, lactation (production of milk) will occur.

PHYSIOLOGY

Production of milk begins within the week following parturition, usually on the third or fourth day in the primagravida. Prior to milk "coming in," the nursing baby receives colostrum, which has been produced throughout the second half of gestation. Factors relating to the amount of colostrum produced are as yet unclear. Milk production or lactation is dependent on multiple factors postpartum, with the pituitary gland having a central role. However, lactation will begin even in the absence of pituitary function (as in women undergoing hypophysectomy during pregnancy, or as in Sheehan's Syndrome, where there is intrapartum infarction of the pituitary) but lactation is not then maintained. The presence of placental lactogen immediately postpartum is believed to be responsible for these observations of early lactation in the absence of the pituitary (3). To maintain lactation, it is necessary to have a normally functioning pituitary gland; to achieve optimal lactation (best milk production) it also is necessary to have normal levels of cortisol, thyroid hormone, parathyroid hormone, and insulin (1,2).

Maintenance of lactation requires the proper functioning of two neuro-endocrine reflexes which involve hormone release from the pituitary. These are [1] the reflex release of prolactin in response to sucking and [2] the "let-down" reflex or milk ejection reflex, mediated by oxytocin.

Prolactin Release

During pregnancy the pituitary increases up to 50 per cent in size and volume. This reflects proliferation of prolactin-producing cells within the anterior pituitary. Throughout pregnancy there is a steady rise in maternal prolactin levels from about 10 ng/ml prepregnancy to about 200 ng/ml at term, or an approximate 20-fold increase (2,4) (see Fig. 2-4). The rising level of prolactin during pregnancy is believed to be responsible (in conjunction with placental lactogen, estrogen and progesterone) for differentiation of the acinar cells of the mammary glands into metabolically active cells capable of milk production. The effect of prolactin and placental lactogen to initiate lactation (actual milk production) is believed to be countered by the high levels of estrogen also present during pregnancy (2,3,5). At parturition there is a prompt fall in estrogen, progesterone, and placental lactogen—and initiation of lactation. Prolactin levels also fall, but if nursing occurs, prolactin rises intermittently with suckling, reaching levels of 8 to 10 times basal levels with a slow fall back to baseline during the time between feedings

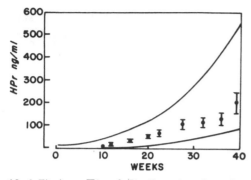

Figure 2-4. Prolactin concentrations.

Basal serum prolactin concentrations between the tenth and fortieth weeks of normal gestation. Selected points represent the mean and the standard error of more than 15 separate determinations. The zone lines represent the wide range of HPr values to be found in pregnancy. (HPr = human prolactin)

From Tysen, JE, Hwang P, Gujda, H, Friesen, HG: Studies of Prolactin Secretion in human Pregnancy. Am J Obstet. Gynecol. 113:14-20, 1972. p. 15.

(2,6,7) (see Fig. 2-5). Levels of prolactin are higher during sleep and at night during lactation (similar to peaks in non-lactating women). Basal levels are somewhat higher in lactating, as compared to non-lactating, postpartum women during the first weeks and months of nursing. The effect of suckling on prolactin release decreases or disappears with time despite continued lactation (2,6,7). Milk production is initiated in the week postpartum even if suckling does not occur but is not maintained without ongoing nursing (or breast pumping).

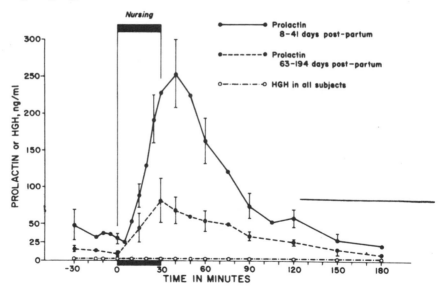

Figure 2-5. Prolactin levels during nursing and breast stimulation. The graph shows plasma prolactin and growth hormone concentrations during nursing in postpartum women. Twelve studies were performed on 8 women between 8 and 41 days postpartum, and six studies were performed on 6 women between 63 and 194 days postpartum. Vertical lines indicate standard error of the mean. Growth hormone, shown at the bottom, did not rise with sucking.

From Noel GL, Sule, HK, Frantz, AG: Prolactin Release During Nursing and Breast Stimulation in Postpartum and Nonpostpartum subjects. J. Clin. Endrocrinol. Metab. 38:413-423, 1974. p. 415.

Prolactin acts directly on the alveolar cells to induce production of milk protein, milk fat, and lactose (2) (see later this chapter).

Milk supply then is dependent on prolactin secretion which occurs in response to suckling. Afferent fibers from the richly innervated nipple and areola are stimulated by suckling (or, to a lesser extent, by expressing milk with a breast pump) (6). The reflex arc travels through spinothalmic tracts to the hypothalamus, where a postulated prolactin-inhibiting factor (PIF) is itself inhibited (2), allowing prolactin secretion by the anterior pituitary. (PIF is postulated because of the observation that in stalk transection of the pituitary, or in lesions destroying hypothalamus, there is a chronic rise in prolactin levels and sometimes galactorrhea.) A positive feedback loop also is possible and may involve thyroid-releasing factor (TRF) which is known to produce a rise in serum prolactin (2,3,5). (This positive loop might explain the occurrence of galactorrhea in some cases of primary hypothyroidism in which elevated levels of TRF occur.) (see Fig. 2-6.)

Milk production is in a steady state with suckling stimulation. The more suckling, the more milk produced (8),this effect apparently mediated by prolactin release. When lactation is successful, there is a continuous feedback between mother and baby with maternal milk supply meeting the baby's suckling "demand." The milk supply is increased when both breasts are offered at each feeding, when nursings are frequent, and when long periods of "milk stasis" are avoided. These factors all relate ultimately to adequate suckling stimulation. The baby's suckling is clearly central to control of the milk supply. The newborn's need for prolonged suckling has the effect of prolonging the period of prolactin secretion and is important in insuring induction and maintenance of an adequate milk supply.

The effect of suckling on prolactin secretion can be partially duplicated by manual or breast pump expression in the pregnant or lactating woman. It also is seen in some non-lactating non-pregnant women who pump their breasts (6) and explains the ability of some women to induce lactation without a recent or previous pregnancy and then to nurse an adopted infant.

The Let-Down Reflex

The second reflex, the let-down, also known as the draught or milk-flow reflex, is well known to the dairy farmer and also was apparent to the ancient Greeks. The origin of The Milky Way is said to have been Juno's milk spurting to the heavens when her infant, Hercules, just put to the breast by his father, Zeus, slipped off the breast—perhaps voluntarily, to avoid the gushing first flow of the let-down.

Like prolactin secretion, the let-down reflex is stimulated by suckling stimulation (1,2,9,10,11). Once lactation is well established, suckling is the main stimulus. However, in addition to suckling, other stimuli also are capable of triggering this reflex, such as a baby's cry, or the sight (or even the

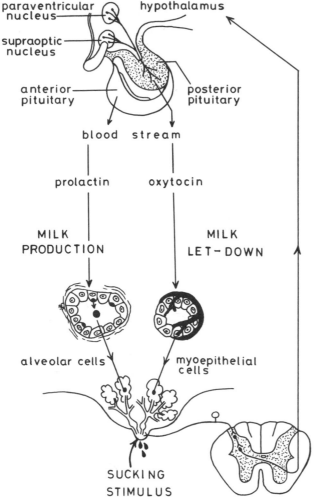

Figure 2-6. Prolactin/oxytocin reflexes. Suckling iniates both reflexes. Prolactin is released from the anterior pituitary when prolactin inhibiting factor is itself inhibited at the level of the hypothalmus. Oxytocin is released from the posterior pituitary where it is stored. It is produced in the nucleus paraventricularis and then transported via nerve axon to the pituitary for storage.

thought) of one's baby. One important cause of failure at breastfeeding is the mother's inability to condition this vital reflex to the baby's nursing. In addition to being stimulated by abstractions (such as the thought of one's baby) the let-down also is easily inhibited during the first days of lactation. Pain, embarrassment, fear, or other sympathetic nervous system stimulation can inhibit the reflex and interfere with normal conditioning to the baby's suckling (2,9).

Suckling stimulation becomes the usual stimulus to the let-down once lactation is well established and is mediated by the afferent fibers from the nipple and areola. The pathway travels through spinothalamic tracts to the hypothalamus and then to the posterior pituitary where oxytocin is released (see Fig. 2-6). Oxytocin is produced in the nucleus paraventricularis in the hypothalamus and is then transported via nerve axons to the posterior pituitary for storage and release. Measurements of oxytocin in the lactating woman show basal levels until the onset of nursing.

Repeated spurts of oxytocin then are released throughout suckling (see Fig. 2-7). Clinically, the nursing mother may be aware of "pins and needles," "a kind of pain," or a "tingling sensation" in the breast which begins shortly after she begins to nurse and disappears gradually (in seconds) after nursing begins (11). Eventually this sensation of the let-down occurs at a set time into each feed, usually within the first minute. It may be accompanied by dripping, or even spurting, of milk from the opposite breast. Should the infant break suction at this point (as did Hercules), gushing streams of milk are seen spurting from the suckled breast. Some women also describe an accompanying sensation of intense thirst that occurs with the let-down. Uterine contractions are also at times felt particularly in multiparas, and

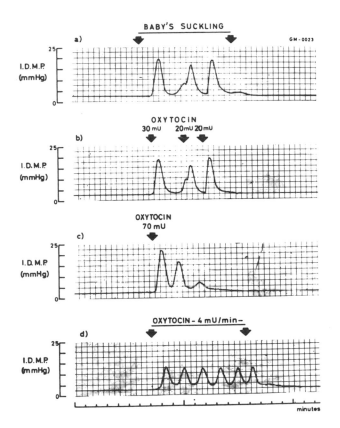

Figure 2-7. Release of oxytocin during suckling. Duplication of the response evoked by suckling. I.D.M.P. = Intraductal mammary pressure. Note that the best duplication of a baby's suckling (a) occurs when oxytocin is given in small spurts as in (b) rather than in a large bolus (c) or continuously (d).

From Cobo E, DeBernal MM, Gaitan E, Quintero, CA: Neurophypophysal hormone release in the human. II Experimental study during lactation. Am J Obstet. Gynecol. 97:519-529, 1967. p. 524.

reflect the sensitivity of the uterine myometrium to oxytocin (10). This correlates clinically with the more rapid involution of the uterus in nursing mothers as compared to those mothers who do not nurse.

The letting down of milk is a result of direct stimulation of the M-E cells by oxytocin. Oxytocin causes contraction of the cells which then pushes the milk that is stored in the distal alveoli and ducts into larger ducts and lactiferous sinuses (beneath the areola). The milk then is available to the nursing baby (1,2). This occurs repeatedly throughout suckling. If the reflex is inhibited the baby is unable to obtain most of the milk present—the stored milk remains in the distal ducts and milk sacs. His sucking can then remove milk only from the central milk sinuses; the reflex is necessary to move the milk from the distal ducts and sacs where it is produced and stored between feeds.

The occurrence of sympathetic inhibition of the let-down reflex appears to be both a direct effect of sympathetic nerves on the M-E cells (inhibiting contraction) and an indirect effect of sympathetic vasoconstriction of mammary vessels (2). Vasoconstriction causes decreased blood flow, and therefore decreased levels of oxytocin reach the breast tissue. This inhibition is sometimes a significant clinical problem during early lactation (the "learning period").

The importance of these reflexes to the clinical management of breastfeeding will be discussed in later sections.

HUMAN MILK AND COLOSTRUM

Colostrum is a clear yellow fluid of higher protein and lower fat and lactose content than either transitional or mature milk. The higher protein content reflects the high concentration of immunoglobulins present, which account for about 95% of the protein in colostrum. In one study, IgA was measured at 12 g% in the first day postpartum (12), a level many times higher than maternal serum values. IgA levels fall to basal levels of about .350 g% by the end of the first week, and eventually continue at about .150 g% (12), ten times maternal serum values (13) (see Fig. 2-8). IgM present at 10% mean maternal serum levels initially falls to about .9% maternal serum levels in mature milk (13); IgG, present in very low levels in colostrum, falls to .3% maternal serum levels (13).

Also recently documented is the presence in colostrum of significant numbers of mononuclear cells. Estimates of the number vary from about 2500 cells/mm^3 to 1-2 X 10^6 cells/mm^3 (14, 15, 16). (Polymorphonuclear cells appear during breast infection and are noted in non-nursing women only irregularly. They are found in low numbers in nursing women (14).) Most of the mononuclear cells (80-90%) are macrophages, which are mobile and which are capable of phagocytosis. The remaining cells are lympho-

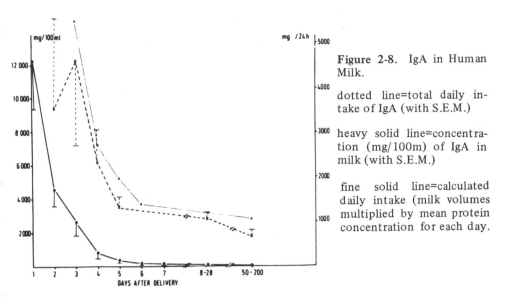

Figure 2-8. IgA in Human Milk.

dotted line=total daily intake of IgA (with S.E.M.)

heavy solid line=concentration (mg/100m) of IgA in milk (with S.E.M.)

fine solid line=calculated daily intake (milk volumes multiplied by mean protein concentration for each day.

Levels of IgA are very high at birth (to 12 g%), fall rapidly during first days. Total quantity of IgA ingested by infant remains significant because of increasing volumes of milk ingested. From McLelland, DBL, McGrata, J. Samson, RR: Antimicrobial factors in human milk. Acta Paedicitr. Scand. Suppl. 271, Sept. 1978. pp. 1-20, p.8.

cytes, which in vitro can be shown to be immunologically active. About half are B and half T lymphocytes. These cells are observed to undergo interaction with colostral macrophages in vitro (14). It can also be demonstrated in vitro that milk lymphocytes can differentiate into plasma cells (16) and that there is synthesis of IgA and β1C by colostral cells; it is postulated that the colostral (and later, milk) lymphocytes are the source of IgA in breast milk (17). In addition to cells and immunoglobulins, the complete complement system as well as factors of the alternate complement pathway can be demonstrated in colostrum and human milk (18).

With transition from colostrum to milk, there is a decrease in the number of cells/mm³ as well as in the concentrations of immunoglobulins present. Total quantity of breast secretion however is increasing during this period, so significant quantities of protein and cells are still ingested by the nursing baby. Over the first four weeks the composition of the milk changes slowly from "transitional" to "mature" milk. That is, there is a gradual increase in fat and lactose content and a fall in protein concentration. Concentrations of sodium, potassium, and chloride also decrease. Calcium and phosphorus concentrations are constant (see Table 2-1).

Mature milk then is achieved by the end of the first month of lactation. At that time chemical studies of milk of various populations of women show that the composition of milk is fairly consistent; levels of protein, fat, and lactose are very similar despite wide variations in maternal diet in various cultures (19). There are, however, variations in specific fatty acid composition (but not in total fat content, which remains constant). Fatty acids present in breast milk generally reflect maternal diet (20). In poorly nourished women, the composition of milk is not significantly altered: concentrations of protein, lactose, and fat are constant. However, total milk yields are lower. In starvation, milk fat reflects the composition of maternal fat stores, and the total milk supply is markedly diminished (19).

Estimates of total quantities of milk produced by well-nourished mothers show a steady increase in quantity from about 600 ml in the first month to about 800 ml in the sixth month. At about that time, as solids are added to the baby's diet, milk supply begins to decrease. However, if nursing continues, maternal milk supply can remain at significant levels and form a significant part of the child's diet past the first year of life.

In discussing the absolute composition of human milk, it is important to remember that there is significant variation in fat composition within each woman's milk during each day and within each feed. "Fore" milk, the first milk expressed during a nursing period, is clear, thin, and bluish, reflecting its low fat and high water content. "Hind" milk, the last milk obtained at the end of a feed, is thick and cream-white, reflecting its higher fat content. Fat content is highest early in the day and lowest at night. The exact composition of the fatty acids, as mentioned, depends on the maternal diet.

Each mammalian milk varies in composition, apparently with the needs of the particular species. There is a rough inverse correlation between rate of growth and protein content in various milks (21). Man, having a slow growth rate, has low protein (.9%); the rat has a fast growth rate and high

---

Note to Table 2-1. Nutrients in Human Breast Milk (Content per Liter of Different Nutrients in Human Breast Milk, Cow's Milk, Evaporated Cow's Milk, Three Proprietary Milks, and Home-Prepared Breast-Milk Substitute).

From Hambraeus, L: Proprietary milk versus human breast milk in infant feeding. A critical appraisal from the nutritional point of view. Pediatric Clinic of North America 24: 17-36, 1977. p. 22.

Studies of breast milk composition are complicated by the difficulty in obtaining adequate specimens.

The variation in fat and protein within a feed, as well as diurnal variations, make small or infrequent specimens inaccurate. The variability of let-down due to emotional factors and the inefficiency of obtaining specimens by pump or hand-expression (as compared to the suckling baby) makes adequate samples difficult to obtain.

Jelliffe's figures do indicate a remarkable consistency of total protein content (0.8-0.9 g%) despite state of maternal nutrition. Range in lactose concentration in various cultures was 6.20-7.67 g% (21).

Table 2-1 Nutrients in Human Breast Milk

	HUMAN BREAST MILK	COW'S MILK	EVAPORATED COW'S MILK	ARTIFICIAL FORMULAS			
				I nonfat milk, vegetable oils, carbohydrate (lactose) (conventional)	II nonfat milk, demineralized whey, vegetable oils, and carbohydrate ("humanized")	III soy flour, vegetable oils, corn syrup and/or sucrose ("milk-free")	IV cow's milk (3% fat), margarine (vegetable fat with 25% C 18:2), corn starch, and sucrose/glucose (home-prepared)
Energy (kcal)	690	660	1520	700	700	700	670
Protein (gm)	9	35	73	15	15	31	17
Fat (gm)	45	37	82	37	36	26-36	25
Carbohydrate (gm)	68	49	106	70	72	52-77	69
lactose (gm)	68	49	106	70	72	–	24
Ash (gm)	2	7	16	4	3	5-8	?
Minerals							
Calcium (mg)	340	1170	2750	536	445	1060-1200	600
Phosphorus (mg)	140	920	2112	454	300	530-800	475
Sodium (mEq)	7	22	55	11	6	10-22	14
Potassium (mEq)	13	35	77	19	14	33-41	21
Chloride (mEq)	11	29	46	12	10	14-16	17
Iron (mg)	0.5	5	22	1.5	13	5-8	0.5
Vitamins							
A (IU)	1898	1025	1850	1650	2650	1590-2110	815
Thiamine (µg)	160	440	280	510	710	530	200
Riboflavin (µg)	360	1750	1900	620	1060	850-1060	900
Niacin (mg)	1.5	0.9	1	9	9	7-9	5
Pyridoxine (µg)	100	640	370	410	420	420	230
Folic acid (µg)	52	55	55	100	32	70	?
B_{12} (µg)	0.3	4	1-2	2	1	2	?
C (mg)	43	11	6	52	58	42-53	8
D (IU)	22	14	420	413	423	420	48
E (IU)	2	0.4	1	12	9	5-11	3
K (µg)	15	60	0-160	–	–	90	80
Examples of products				Enfamil Similac	SMA	Sobee MullSoy	

milk protein (12%). The cow is intermediate in rate of growth and in milk protein content (3.4%). Lactose correlates roughly inversely with protein content. Human milk has among the highest lactose concentrations (about 7% of milk); milk of the rat lower (about 3%); and again, the cow intermediate at about 5% (21). Low protein concentrations also correlate with species that require frequent feeds (continuous feeding species) and high protein with species that feed infrequently (19).

Human milk then is about 50% fat, .9% protein, and 7% lactose. Its total nitrogen content of 1.2% is now known to include a significant portion of non-protein nitrogen (21).

When milk protein is digested in the stomach of the newborn, it is separated into two fractions [1] casein, a Ca^{++}-phosphorus-containing precipitate, and [2] whey proteins, those proteins which remain in solution. In human milk, the ratio of whey proteins to casein is about 70:20. The whey proteins of human milk consist mostly of a-lactalbumin (40% of the total protein) and lactoferrin (25%). In addition there are small amounts of other proteins: lysozyme (.08%), albumin (.08%), IgA, IgG, IgM (.16%). Non-protein nitrogen, about ¼ of total nitrogen present, includes urea nitrogen, creatine nitrogen, uric acid, glucosamine, a-amino nitrogen, ammonia nitrogen, and other as yet unidentified components (21) (see Table 2-2)

In comparison, cow's milk protein has a whey-to-casein ratio of about 20:80. Cow's milk whey is mostly β-lactoglobulin, a protein not present in human milk, with only small amounts of a-lactalbumin and traces of lactoferrin, the main proteins of human milk.

The casein of human milk is distinct from that of all other mammalian species in its amino acid composition. It has a very low ratio of methionine: cystine, as compared to that of other animal proteins, reflecting its very high cystine and low methionine concentration (22). It is of note that cystathionase, necessary in the conversion of methionine to cystine, is not present in the premature infant. Cystine, then, is an essential amino acid for the prematurely born newborn. Breast milk also contains much lower levels of phenylanine and tyrosine (aromatic amino acid) than other mammalian milks (22).

The curd of the breastfed human infant is softer, smaller, and sweeter smelling than that of the formula-fed infant. Digestion of human milk protein is more efficient and faster, and absorption is more complete than that of cow's-milk protein.

The composition of human milk fat vs. cow's milk fat also is different: long-chain unsaturated fatty acids and polyunsaturated fatty acids predominate in human milk, while saturated fatty acids are mainly found in cow's

Table 2-2

Protein Nitrogen and Nonprotein Nitrogen
in Human Milk and Cow's Milk
(Values refer to gm N per liter; values within brackets
refer to gm protein per liter)

	HUMAN MILK		COW'S MILK	
Total nitrogen	1.93		5.31	
Protein nitrogen	1.43 (8.9)		5.03 (31.4)	
Casein nitrogen		0.40 (2.5)		4.37 (27.3)
Whey protein nitrogen		1.03 (6.4)		0.93 (5.8)
α-lactalbumin		0.42 (2.6)		0.17 (1.1)
lactoferrin		0.27 (1.7)		traces
β-lactoglobulin		–		0.57 (3.6)
lysozyme		0.08 (0.5)		traces
serum albumin		0.08 (0.5)		0.07 (0.4)
Ig A		0.16 (1.0)		0.005 (0.03)
Ig G		0.005 (0.03)		0.096 (0.6)
Ig M		0.003 (0.02)		0.005 (0.03)
Nonprotein nitrogen	0.50		0.28	
Urea nitrogen	0.25		0.13	
Creatine nitrogen	0.037		0.009	
Creatinine nitrogen	0.035		0.003	
Uric acid nitrogen	0.005		0.008	
Glucosamine	0.047		?	
α-amino nitrogen	0.13		0.048	
Ammonia nitrogen	0.002		0.006	
Nitrogen from other components	?		0.074	

From Hambraeus, L: Proprietary milk versus human breast milk in infant feeding. A critical appraisal from the nutritional point of view. Pediatric Clinic of North America 24: 17-36, 1977. Pg. 21, after Forsum, E and Lönnerdal B: Protein evaluation of breast mik substitutes with special reference to the nonprotein nitrogen (unpublished data).

milk (21). Breast milk contains a bile-salt stimulated lipase, capable of rapid digestion of human milk fat. This lipase, in addition to the specificity of the fatty acids present in human milk may account for the more efficient digestion and absorption of human milk fat (23). There is no loss of fat in the stools of the breastfed infant; significant losses occur with cow's milk formula feeds (24). (Many modern formulas use vegetable oils and medium chain tryglycerides in place of cow's milk fat in an attempt to decrease this loss (21) (see Table 2-3).

Lactose is the main carbohydrate and is about 7% of human milk vs. 4.8% of cow's milk, giving breast milk its sweeter taste. (Formulas have added lactose or other carbohydrate to approximate human milk sugar content.) Another carbohydrate, the "bifidus factor," is one of a group of nitrogen containing complex carbohydrates found in human milk (see Chapter 4.)

Mineral and electrolyte concentrations in breast milk are lower than in cow's milk (25):

	sodium	potassium	calcium	phosphorus	ratio of Ca/p
human milk:	7mEq/L	13 mEq/L	340 mg/L	140 mg/L	2/1
cow's milk:	20	35	1170	920	1.3/1

Table 2-3

Fatty Acid Content in Human Breast Milk, Cow's Milk and
Two Types of Proprietary Milks
(Values are given as gm per 100 gm fat)

FATTY ACID	HUMAN MILK	COW'S MILK	SMA	SIMILAC
Saturated				
C 10:0	1.0	2.4	1.4	2.1
C 12:0	4.8	3.2	14.5	18.7
C 14:0	6.2	11.5	6.0	7.3
C 16:0	23.7	30.0	12.8	9.4
C 18:0	6.7	14.3	7.4	3.1
Unsaturated				
C 16:1	4.6	2.0	1.0	trace
C 18:1	37.4	31.1	38.9	19.2
C 18:2	9.0	1.8	13.1	40.2
C 18:3	3.4	trace	1.1	trace

*From Widdowson, E. M., Southgate, D. A. T., and Schutz, Y.: Comparison of dried milk preparations for babies on sale in 7 European countries. I. Protein, fat, carbohydrate and inorganic constituents. Arch. Dis. Child., 49:867, 1974, with permission.

No formula exactly duplicates the chemical content of breast milk. The formula PM 60/40 attains a similar electrolyte content to that of human milk, but has higher protein content. The formula SMA has a low (1.5 g%) protein content but the ratio Ca/P is 1.3. The lower electrolyte concentrations of breast milk ensure that sufficient free water is available to the infant. The fully nursing normal infant requires no extra water even in tropical heat or with febrile illness. (The breastfed infant with severe diarrheal disease may become hypotonically dehydrated, unlike the bottle-fed infant in whom hypertonicity and acidosis in similar circumstances is common.) (26) The ratio of Ca/P of 2.1 (the ratio in human milk) is sought by the makers of infant formulas because of the incidence of neonatal hypocalcemia in some infants who are fed cow's milk formula with lower ratios.

By definition, the concentration of vitamins, trace substances, and minerals present in breast milk of well-fed mothers are often taken to represent optimal standards for infant nutrition. Questions about the adequacy of iron and vitamin D content of human milk, however, have been raised and are discussed below. Clearly, other vitamins and trace minerals (and perhaps as yet unrecognized factors) are in sufficient concentration if mother is adequately nourished. Deficiencies of any and all vitamins occur, however, if the mother is seriously deficient. Maternal stores are depleted in order to maintain normal levels in breastmilk. Once maternal stores are depleted, deficiencies will occur in milk. The iron deficient mother may have decreased iron concentrations in her milk. The vegetarian who eats no milk, eggs, fish or meat is at risk herself for B_{12} deficiency and eventually for a deficiency in her milk and therefore in her breastfed infant.

Iron deficiency is rare in term born breastfed infants of well nourished women. Despite this, the practice of giving iron supplements to breastfed children has been common. This practice reflects the frequency of iron deficiency in formula-fed infants and the known low iron content of human milk. However, despite its low iron content, the iron present in human milk is better absorbed than the iron present in formula or cow's milk (27, 28). Totally breastfed infants can triple their birthweight, maintaining normal iron status without iron supplements (29). Once solids are started, at four to six months, extra sources of iron may be needed (30). This increased requirement possibly reflects interference with absorption of milk iron once solids are added to the diet. Ideally, then, a full term infant of a well-nourished mother needs no iron supplementation or solid foods to maintain iron status until he begins solids and/or triples his birthweight. At that time, foods rich in iron can be started, avoiding any need for medicinal iron.*

The premature infant is born with insufficient iron stores and should be followed closely for iron deficiency. The need for iron supplementation is likely to occur early, and routine prescription of iron supplementation may be appropriate.

The occurrence of rickets in breastfed infants is unusual but has been reported (At present cow's milk and formulas are all vitamin D fortified). Recently a water soluble vitamin D sulfate has been isolated and measured in human milk and may explain the adequacy of breast milk in preventing rickets (31). Previously, measured vitamin D levels in breast milk (.01 mg/dl or .42 U.S.P. units) reflected measurement only of the fat soluble vitamin (1). Levels of 1.00 mg/dl of the vitamin D sulfate have been meas-

---

*Fomon, S.J. et al. (Pediatrics 63:52, 1979) continue to recommend routine iron supplementation of all breastfed infants, believing that even with optimal absorption the quantity of iron available in breast milk is insufficient. Further clinical study is clearly needed to clarify this issue. No scientific evidence supports Fomon's statement.

ured in breast milk and may represent adequate doses (31). However, the physiological role of this new vitamin D is not yet studied, nor are the factors which control its levels in breast milk. Therefore, at present it is safer to prescribe vitamin D to breastfed infants who will not be exposed to sunlight (400 IU vitamin D/day).

Breastfed infants, like bottle-fed infants, should routinely be given vitamin K at birth as prophylaxis against hemmorhagic disease of the newborn (1 mg vitamin K-1 I.M. or p.o.), as adequate levels of the vitamin depend on gut flora not present at birth (32).

References

1. Kon, SK and Cowie, AT: *Milk: The Mammary Gland and Its Secretions.* New York: Academic Press, 1961.

2. Vorherr, H: *The Breast.* New York: Academic Press, 1974.

3. Josimovich, JB, ed.: *Lactogenic Hormones, Fetal Nutrition and Lactation.* USA: John Wiley & Sons, Inc., 1974.

4. Tyson, JE, Hwang, P, et al.: Studies of prolactin secretion in human pregnancy. Am. J. Obstet. Gynecol. 113:14, 1972.

5. Tyson, JE, Khojcendi, M, et al.: The influence of prolactin secretion on human lactation. J. Clin. Endocrinol. Metab. 40:764, 1975.

6. Noel, GL, Suh, HK et al: Prolactin release during nursing and breast pump stimulation in postpartum and nonpostpartum subjects. J. Clin. Endocrinol. Metab. 38:413, 1974.

7. Bunner, DL, VanderLaan, EF, VanderLaan, WP: Prolactin levels in nursing mothers. Am. J. Obstet. Gynecol. 131:250, 1978.

8. Egli, GE, Egli, NS and Newton, H: Influence of the number of breastfeedings on milk production. Pediatrics 27:314, 1961.

9. Newton, M, Newton, N: The let-down reflex in human lactation. J. Pediatr. 33:698, 1948.

10. Caldeyro-Barcia, M. and Folley, SJ, eds: Milk Ejection in Women, in Reynolds, M, *Lactogenesis.* Philadelphia: U. of Penn. Press, 1969, p. 229.

11. Ibister, C: A clinical study of the draught reflex in human lactation. Arch. Dis. Child. 29:66, 1954.

12. McClelland, DBL, McGrath, J, Samson, R: Antimicrobial factors in human milk. Acta Paediatr. Scand. Supplement 271, 1978.

13. Goldman, AS: Immunological aspects of breastfeeding. La Leche League Convention, October 20, 1978. (6th annual seminar on breastfeeding for physicians.)

14. Smith, CW, and Goldman, AS: The cells of human colostrum. Pediatr. Res. 2:103, 1968.

15. Lawton and Shortbridge: Protective factors in human breast milk and colostrum. Lancet 1: 253, 1957.

16. Pitt, J: Breast milk leukocytes. Pediatr. 58:769, 1976.

17. Murillo, G.J. and Goldman, AS: The cells of human colostrum. Pediatr. Res. 4:71, 1970.

18. Nakajima, S: Complement system in human colostrum. Int. Archs. Allergy Appl. Immunol. 54:428, 1977.

19. Jelliffe, D and Jelliffe, EFP: *Human Milk in the Modern World.* Oxford: Oxford Univ. Press, 1978.

20. Insell, W, Jr, et al.: The fatty acids of human milk. J. Clin. Invest. 38:443, 1959.

21. Hambraeus, L: Proprietary milk versus human milk in infant feeding: a critical appraisal from the nutritional point of view. Pediatr. Clin. N.A. 24:17, 1977.

22. Gyorgy, P: Biochemical aspects from the uniqueness of human milk. Am. J. Clin. Nutr. 24:970, 1971.

23. Hernell, O et al.: Breast milk composition in Ethiopian and Swedish mothers, IV. Milk lipases. Am. J. Clin. Nutr. 30:508, 1977.

24. Fomon, SJ et at.: Excretion of fat by normal full-term infants fed various milks and formulas. Amer. J. Clin. Nutr. 23:1299, 1970.

25. Fomon, SJ: *Infant Nutrition.* Philadelphia: W.B. Saunders, 1974.

26. Kingston, M: Biochemical disturbances in breastfed infants with gastroenteritis. J. Pediatr. 82:1073, 1973.

27. McMillan, J. et al.: Iron absorption from human milk. Pediatrics 60:896, 1977.

28. Saarinen, V.M., et al.: Iron absorption in infants. J. Pediatr. 91:36, 1977.

29. McMillan, J, et al.: Iron sufficiency in breast-fed infants. Pediatrics 58:686, 1976.

30. Saarinen, VM: Need for iron supplementation in infants on prolonged breastfeeding. J. Pediatr. 93:177, 1978.

31. Lakdawala, DR and Widdowson, EM: Vitamin D in human milk. Lancet 1:167, 1977.

32. Rudolph, AM: *Pediatrics*. New York: Appleton-Century-Crofts, 1977.

Chapter 3

The Pharmacology of Drugs And Chemicals in Human Milk

by
Cheston M. Berlin, Jr., M.D.

Professor of Pediatrics
Professor of Pharmacology
The Pennsylvania State University College of Medicine
Hershey, Pennyslvania, 17033

The composition of human breast milk has not been surpassed for feeding infants. The many advantages have been summarized in several publications (1-4), and are discussed in the next chapter.

The recent increase in breastfeeding is occurring at a time of continuing drug use, both prescription and over-the-counter. It is well known that many (indeed, perhaps all) drug and environmental chemicals are transferred from maternal plasma to milk. Most studies have measured the concentration of a drug in milk at only a single time point after maternal dosing. Simultaneous levels in maternal plasma or saliva are frequently not measured.

It must be emphasized that virtually all work on breast function/milk secretion has been done in animal species. The difficulty of studying human lactation (anatomically and physiologically) using current methods of continuous milk collection, serial biopsy of lactating tissue, and administration of isotopic biochemical precursors, is obvious. But, there is no reason to suppose the formation of human milk is fundamentally different from other animal studies.

A way of summarizing what has been said about the anatomy of the lactating breast is that it resembles a bunch of grapes, with each grape being tear-shaped and consisting of a cluster of alveolar cells in which breast milk is synthesized and secreted into a central lumen. The lumens feed into small ducts that meet each other in channels of increasing size until the nipple region is reached. With the possible exception of water transport, little alteration in the composition of the milk occurs once it leaves the alveolar lumen. Excretion of drugs into milk most likely occurs only within this lumen.

Human milk is a suspension of fat and protein in a carbohydrate (lactose) - mineral solution. A nursing mother will easily produce 1 liter of milk per day (amount needed to provide ample nourishment for a 6.7 kg infant) containing 9 g of protein,* 36 g of fat and 72 g of lactose with the correct amount of minerals and most vitamins. Human milk also contains a number of substances which protect the infant from infection, immunoglobulins, macrophages, lymphocytes, transferrin, lactoferrin, interferon, complement, and nonprotein nitrogen. The exact composition of human milk varies with duration of lactation and may even vary within a single feeding. There is a definite need for modern data on the composition of human milk.

Milk protein is synthesized entirely within the mammary gland. A small amount of plasma protein does enter into breast milk, presumably across the alveolar cell and/or through extracellular space between these cells. The major proteins are casein and lactalbumin (latter also needed for lactose synthesis). Synthesis is initiated by prolactin and needs insulin and hydrocortisone to continue. The proteins are very digestible and contribute to the low curd-tension of human milk. Proteins are transported from the endoplasmic reticulum into the Golgi apparatus, migrate from the base of the cell towards the apex, and are discharged into the alveolar lumen via apocrine secretion. The role of these proteins in binding drugs has yet to be completely investigated. In the two reported studies that specifically measured drug (theobromine and theophylline) binding to human milk protein, it was found to vary between 0% and 24% (5,6).

Short-chain fatty acids are synthesized in the mammary gland from acetate. Long-chain fatty acids are transferred from plasma. Both classes of fat are esterified in the breast with glycerol (derived from intracellular glucose). The lipids collect in the endoplasmic reticulum. As they ascend the cell in ever-increasing droplets they acquire a three layered membrane (lipoprotein) and are extruded into milk as milk-fat globules (7). It is intriguing to speculate on the possibilities of drug binding to both the protein and fat component of the milk-fat globule. It is also possible that

* This figure is disputed. (See Chapter 2)

some lipid-soluble drugs may be trapped entirely within the milk-fat globule.

Lactose is entirely synthesized in the breast alveolar cell. Its synthesis proceeds from UDP-galactose and glucose with lactose synthetase (galactose-transferase plus lactalbumin) as the enzyme. Prolactin is absolutely required. Lactose is excreted from the cell into the alveolar lumen alone and with milk protein.

Electrolytes, vitamin, and water are supplied by the cell (from plasma water) to achieve the final concentration.

All of the above elements achieve a concentration in human milk which provides the ideal nutrient supply to the infant for at least the first 6 months. After 6 months the infant's caloric need usually requires supplemental food.

The transport of drugs into breast milk from maternal tissues and plasma may proceed by a number of routes.

Figure 3-1 is a schematic drawing of the alveolar breast cell and illustrates the cellular structures that a substance in maternal plasma must traverse to enter milk contained within the alveolar lumen. After crossing the capillary endothelium, the drug traverses the interstitular space and must cross the basement membrane (mostly mucopolysaccharides) of the alveolar breast cell. The cell plasma membrane is trilaminar with the usual phospholipid-protein membrane structure. After reaching the cell cytoplasm the compound travels apically and leaves the cell by diffusion, reverse pinocytosis, or apocrine secretion (the apical part of the cell disintegrates). This entire process is nicely detailed by Vorherr (8). The following are the most probable mechanisms of drug excretion in milk:

. . . . .Mechanisms of Drug Excretion in Milk . . . .

1.   *Transcellular diffusion.* Small unionized molecules with liquid solubility such as urea and ethanol transverse the capillary epithelium, intercellular water, basal cell membrane, and the alveolar cell and its apical membrane by diffusion. This mechanism is supported by the observation that milk levels mirror simultaneous plasma levels and the elimination rate constants (calculated from the phase) are similar (9). Compounds with molecular weights under 200 diffuse best.

2.   *Intercellular diffusion.* This route avoids the breast alveolar cell entirely. Histological studies in some animal species suggest that such a space may not exist or is very tight (see Fig. 3-1). It may be important functionally in the human and may explain how large molecules such as interferon and immunoglobulins enter human milk.

3.   Small ionized molecules and small proteins may enter the basal part of the cell from interstitial water through *passive diffusion in water-filled channels.* Molecular weight also is limiting here (less than 200 diffuses best).

4.   Polar substances may penetrate by being bound to *carrier proteins* with cell membrane (ionophore diffusion).

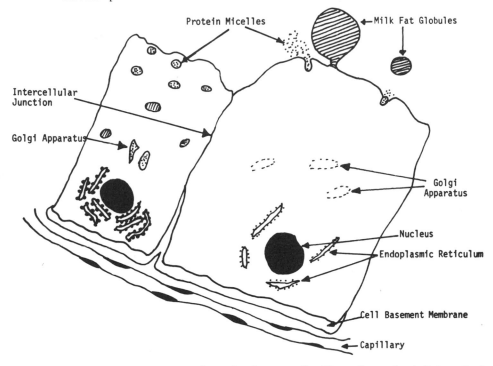

Figure 3-1. Schematic drawing of aveolar breast cells. The cell on the left is actively synthesizing protein, fat, and carbohydrate. The cell on the right has discharged most of the products into the alveolar lumen as milk. Carbohydrate is secreted with protein.

Diffusion appears to be the most common mechanism for a drug to cross a cell membrane. The distribution of a drug across a lipid biological membrane has been shown to depend on the degree of ionization of the drug plus the assumption that a pH difference exists across the membrane—it is the unionized fraction that diffuses through the membrane (10). Knowing the degree of ionization of the drug (pK_a) plus the pH difference, the theoretical milk/plasma (M/P) ratio can be calculated.* Figure 3-2 illus-

* Acknowledgement must be made to the elegant experiments by Dr. Rasmussen in defining this process in the animal models of the lactating cow and goat. He has a very clear and significant discussion in reference 11.

trates the situation for 2 weakly acidic drugs with markedly different pK_a's: salicylic acid (pK_a=3.0) and phenobarbital (pK_a=7.2). Plasma pH is assumed to be 7.4 and milk pH 7.0 (commonly accepted for human milk). For a weak acid the Henderson-Hasselbach equation defines the ratio of unionized to ionized drug (at equilibrium) as:

$$\log \frac{U}{I} = pK_a - pH$$

$$\text{For a weak base:} \quad \log \frac{I}{U} = pK_a - pH$$

Theoretical M/P ratio for total salicylate (unionized plus ionized) is 0.40; the experimental value obtained by Miller et al. (12) is 0.35. The theoretical ratio for total phenobarbital is 0.46; the experimental value is 0.7 (Rasmussen). This difference for phenobarbital may be explained by the significant lipid-solubility of this drug (chloroform/water distribution

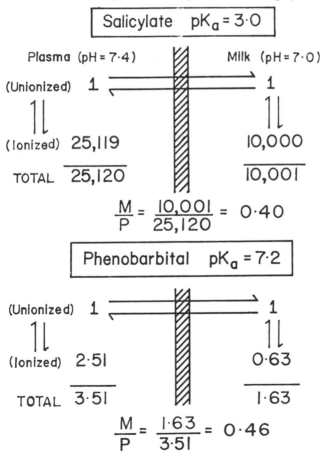

Figure 3-2. Theoretical distribution of weakly acidic drugs across a lipid cell membrane. Units are arbitrary for illustration.

of unionized drug = 4.8). Thus the presence on one side of a biological membrane of a substance rich in fat (milk) will introduce another factor in the final determination of the concentration of a drug in breast milk.

Milk also has .9 g% of protein-which may also bind drugs. Little data is yet available, but Rasmussen has demonstrated sulfonamide binding in milk to be present from 0%-40% depending on the sulfonamide (14).

As a general statement, weak acids (e.g. sulfanilamide, phenobarbital, salicylate, penicillin) will have an M/P ratio (both theoretical and experimental) of less than 1.0. Weak bases (antipyrine, lincomycin, quinine, ephedrine) will have an M/P ratio greater than 1.0 (11). The precise experimental value will depend on factors such as maternal dosing intervals, milk pH , protein binding in plasma and milk, and lipid-solubility of the drug.

The ratio of drug in the ultrafiltrate of milk to that in the ultrafiltrate in plasma was found to be independent of plasma levels (M/P identical at all levels of plasma concentration). The concentration in milk was found also to be constant regardless of volume of milk in the mammary gland. These observations (11) support the thesis that diffusion is the major mechanism for the appearance of drugs in breast milk.

A number of reviews (15-20) give tables of the concentration of drugs in breast milk. Most of these values consist of a single measurement of the drug concentration; the period of time from maternal ingestion is usually not defined nor is maternal dose, frequency of dose, frequency of nursing and length of lactation. Measurement of the drug in the nursing infant's blood or urine is not mentioned. Hence it is not usually possible to determine risk to the nursling with a single isolated point. Many of the quoted references refer to data from the 1940's and 1950's when analytic methods were primitive. For example, the oft-quoted reference (21) to salicylates dates from 1935 and employed a semi-quantitative method ($FeCl_3$) for salicylate analysis; no quantitative values were given. Many of the currently used maternal medications, especially cardiovascular, corticosteroid, and CNS drugs also need precise measurements. The discipline of pharmacokinetics was not developed when many of the drugs in breast milk were assayed. Hence very few detailed studies employing drug measurements over a period of time in both maternal and infant body fluids are available.

There are several other critical questions. What dose does the infant absorb (as measured by infant blood and urine levels) and does the breast excrete any metabolites of the parent drug? Is mammary tissue, which is so metabolically active, itself capable of drug biotransformation?

Table 3-1 is an attempt to list those drugs appearing in milk for which some pharmacokinetic data can be found. The blank spaces in this table cannot be filled using current data. The rather small number of drugs in this table emphasizes the paucity of current knowledge in precisely determining

Table 3-1

Drugs Appearing in Human Milk
for Which Some Pharmacokinetic Data Can Be Found

Drug (reference)	Maternal Dose	ug/ml Peak Level	M/P * Ratio at Peak
Antipyrine (22)	18 mg/kg	20-30	1.0
Cefazolin (23)	2 gm I.V. 500 mg I.M. t.i.d.	1.51 0	0.023
Chlorothiazide (24)	500 mg p.o. Single dose		
Diazepam (25)	Not stated	0.27	0.68
Digoxin (26)	0.25 mg	0.6-1.0 ng/ml	.8-.9
Ethanol (9)	0.6 g/kg	777	0.93
Isoniazid (27)	300 mg	16.6	1.6
Lithium (28)	Chronic; dose not specified	0.1-0.6 mmol/l	0.5
Methadone (29)	70 mg/day	0.36 0.51	0.83 1.89
Nicotine (30)	1 pack/day (400 mg)	91 ng/ml Range 20-512	
Prednisolone (31)	5 mg	26 ng/ml	
Prednisone (32)	120 mg	154 ng/ml (Prednisone) 473 ng/ml (Prednisolone)	
Propranolol (33)	20 mg 160 mg	10 ng/ml 150 ng/ml	.56 .65
Salicylate (34)	20 mg/kg		
Sulphasalazine (35)	2 gms/day (chronic)	9-15 mg/ml (as sulfapyridine)	0.6
Sulphone (36)		14	0.16
Theophylline (6)	4.25 mg/kg	4 ug/ml	0.7

*   M/P = milk/plasma

Time of Peak Level	$t_{1/2}$ **	Amt. Secreted in 24° After Single Dose ***	% Maternal Dose ****
10 min.	6-22 hrs.	7-25 mg	0.5-2.4
3 hrs.		1.5 mg	0.075
Not detected in milk		0	
Not detected in milk (<1 ug/ml)		<1 mg/day	
3 days	3 days	0.27 mg (peak) on on day 3	
4 hrs.	12 hrs.	.18-.36 ug/day	0.07-0.14
90 min.	2.9 hrs.	300 mg	1
3 hrs.	5.9 hrs.	7 mg	2.3
Levels fairly constant			
		300 ug	0.4
No correlation		0.68 mg	0.17
1 hr.	8.2 hrs.	6 ug	0.12
2 hr.	1.8 hrs.	47 ug (as both Prednisone and	0.04
2 hr.	1.1 hrs.	Prednisolone)	
3 hrs.		0.6 ug	0.03
3 hrs.		90 ug	0.05
			0.18-0.36
Constant level		1.4-2.1 mg	0.16
6 hrs.		10 mg	2
2 hrs.	4.0 hrs.	8 mg	4

** $t_{1/2}$ is calculated from the elimination (β) phase.

*** Amount secreted in 24 hours is estimated by assuming the infant ingests 90 cc of milk every 4 hours.

**** The % of maternal dose is calculated by dividing the amount secreted in 24 hours by the maternal dose (single dose or 24 hour maternal dose).

the risk to the nursing infant. The following general points may be made:

1. Most drugs (and environmental chemicals) can cross from plasma to milk.
2. Levels in milk parallel plasma levels in time. Milk/plasma ratios usually vary from 0.5 to 1.0.
3. Following a single maternal dose, $t_{1/2}$ (half life) are similar for plasma and milk. This implies rather rapid transport from plasma to milk (according to M/P ratios).
4. The total amount available for infant absorption is usually less than 1% of maternal dose. This amount may be minimized by planning nursing periods at times of low maternal plasma levels (e.g., just before a maternal dose).
5. Virtually nothing is known about the situation with repetitive maternal doses over days or weeks.
6. For most drugs, even those with potent pharmacologic actions, the risk to the infant, with attention to proper nursing schedule to minimize drug exposure of the infant, is negligible.

For specific drugs not mentioned in this table, the references by Knowles (15) and O'Brien (19) should be consulted.

Table 3-2 lists those few drugs that are contraindicated (or during therapy, nursing is contraindicated) during lactation. The number is small; no doubt it might be increased as more data is collected and with the introduction of new drugs.

The use of radioactive isotopes for diagnostic purposes is very common; all women in the child bearing age should be asked whether they are nursing before an isotope is given. It may be possible to delay the test, employ an alternate test, or give specific instructions of how long to avoid nursing to insure disappearance from milk of all significant radioactivity. Table 3-3 summarizes the excretion of the more commonly used radiopharmaceuticals in human milk. For [99]technetium it is safe to resume nursing after 48 hrs from maternal injection. For [67]gallium or [131]iodine, nursing will usually have to be terminated since it is unlikely that the mother can continue to express by hand (or by breast pump) milk for the 7-14 days necessary to achieve a negligible radiation level in her milk.

ENVIRONMENTAL CHEMICALS

In 1951 Laug et al. (38) published a report of DDT excretion in human-milk samples collected in the United States (Washington, D.C.). They found DDT present in 94% of samples, with a mean level of 0.13 ppm (mg/kg milk).

Table 3-2
Drugs Contraindicated in the Nursing Mother

Drug (reference)	Reason
Lithium (28)	Significant blood levels in the infant (1/3–1/2 maternal levels)
INH (27)	Anti-DNA drug; metabolite (acetyl INH) which is thought responsible for liver toxicity also secreted in milk
Antimetabolites (37)	Anti-DNA activity
Radioactive pharmaceuticals (38,39,40)	Radioactivity present in breast milk (see Table III)
Very lipid soluble drugs (38,39,40,41) (hexachlorophene, PBC's, DDT, THC)	Only elimination route through milk; measure level if any doubt of maternal body burden
Phenindione (56)	Bleeding in one case report with ↑PT and ↑PTT
Mothers homozygous for cystic fibrosis (57)	Sodium content of milk high: 132–280 mEq/l
Chloramphenicol	Possible bone marrow depression
Propylthiouracil	Possible goiter and bone marrow suppression

This is in excess of the level permitted by WHO (39) and the U.S. Code of Federal Regulations (Title 21: 120.147C) of 0.05 ppm. Similar numbers have been reported from other parts of the world including Norway (40,41), Australia (42), the Netherlands (43), and Canada (44). Within the United States similar concentrations of DDT are present in human milk regardless of geographical location or population size (45). In 1951 in the U.S. the amount of DDT found by Laug et al. was 0.13 ppm (38); in Quinby et al. (45) found levels of 0.12 ppm; and in 1972 Kroger (46) found levels of 0.10 ppm from 6 areas throughout the U.S. Mean control of DDT was 0.17 ppm. Thus in the USA, there has been no change in content over 20 years. In Norway 7 years after the total ban on DDT (1969-1970) the level in milk in Oslo had fallen from a mean of .082 ppm in 1969 to 0.050 ppm in 1976 (41). Other areas of Norway showed similar decreases. No decrease was found in the content of other organochlorine compounds (polychlorinated biphenyls, hexachlorobenzene); in fact, there was a significant increase (doubling) in the content of PCBs from 0.011 ppm in 1969 to 0.024 ppm in 1976 (41). There is no evidence that the organochlorines in these concentrations adversely affect nursing infants.

These studies above present information that suggests that these highly lipid-soluble chemicals are stored in body fat and that milk may be the only route of elimination from the body: [1] DDT concentrations are eleven-fold higher in fat samples than milk [2] DDT concentrations decrease with

Table 3-3

Secretion of Radioactive Isotopes in Milk

Isotope (reference)	Maternal Dose	$t\frac{1}{2}$	Amount in Milk Ci/ml	Infant Dose Ci/day	Cumulative Dose to Infant Ci
67Gallium (58)	3 mCi IC	78 hrs	3 days 0.15 7 days 0.045 14 days 0.010	75 23 5	350 (if nursed from day 3 on) 108 (if nursed from day 7 on) 23 (if nursed from day 14 on)
131Iodine (59)	200 µCi IV	24 hrs	25 hrs .028	6	15 (if nursed through day 5) 7.5% of maternal dose
99Technetium (60)	15 mCi IV	4 hrs	8.5 hrs 0.1 20 hrs 0.02 60 hrs 0.006	95	0.63% of maternal dose

The data in the last two columns are calculated by assuming the infant takes 3 ounces of breast milk every four hours.

number of infants nursed [3] DDT concentrations decrease with number of months nursed and, finally [4] DDT concentrations are significantly lower in the end of a single feed.

The unfortunate contamination of cattle feed with polybrominated biphenyls (PBB) on Michigan cattle farms in 1973-1974 resulted in detectable levels of PBB in human milk. For samples from the lower Michigan peninsula (site of the heaviest contamination), 96% were positive for PBB in the range of 0.02-1.0 ppm. The upper peninsula samples were positive for PBB in 43% of samples in a range from 0.02 to 0.5 ppm with most samples below 0.1 (47). There was a high degree of correlation between values in paired samples of milk and adipose tissue. The degree of risk even at these levels is not known.

Other highly lipid soluble chemicals (e.g. tetrahydrocannabinol) may be expected to act in a similar fashion. For women known to have had high exposure (by occupation or food ingestion), it is reasonable to assay milk samples to determine exact risk.

ORAL CONTRACEPTIVES

The widespread postpartum use of oral contraceptive to nursing mothers represents probably the most common drug exposure. Vorherr (48) has summarized 18 separate papers published over 10 years dealing with this problem. It does not appear, using this information, that these compounds significantly interfere with milk production, especially if the contraceptive is withheld for several weeks, until lactation is firmly established.

DRUG METABOLISM IN BREAST TISSUE

Little evidence is available concerning the actual drug metabolizing activity of breast tissue. Rasmussen and Linzell (49) have described the acetylation of sulfanilamide by the mammary tissue of the lactating goat. Dao (50) was unable to demonstrate metabolism of the carcinogen 3-methylcholanthrene in mammary tissue. Bruder et al. (51) have described cytochrome P-420 and cytochrome b_5 in the membranes of the milk fat globule of human milk; the same cytochromes were identified in the rough endoplasmic reticulum of lactating bovine and rat mammary epithelial cells. No cytochrome P-450 was identified in human, bovine or rat milk or mammary tissue. Liu et al. (52) have recently identified a calcium-stimulated ribonuclease in rat milk and mammary tissue. This ribonuclease also has been observed in human milk (53,54). It is intriguing to speculate on its role in light of the observation by Scholm et al. (55) that human milk contains high molecular weight RNA particles.

SUMMARY

Nearly all drugs (or environmental chemicals) may be found in breast milk after maternal ingestion. It is prudent to minimize maternal exposure although very few are known to be hazardous to the nursing infant (see Table 3-2 and Table 3-3). Chronic maternal drug administratión and exposure to high levels of environmental chemicals are areas that need further exploration. More sensitive analytic techniques need to be used to detect metabolites which may present a greater risk than the parent compound. (Breast milk, the ideal infant food, must be made as safe as possible.)

The following are specific suggestions to minimize risk to the nursing infant:

Minimizing Drug Risk
. . . . to the Nursing Infant. . . . .

1.   Avoid maternal drugs whenever possible

2.   Should a nursing mother need a medication, nurse the infant just *before* each dose.

3.   If published information is inadequate to determine concentration in milk, measure the drug in several samples at different time intervals after a test dose. This will not only quantitate the drug, but also will suggest appropriate nursing intervals.

References

1.   Nutrition Committee of the Canadian Paediatric Society and the Committee on Nutrition of the American Academy of Pediatrics: Breast Feeding. Pediatrics 62:591-601, 1978.

2.   Fomon SJ: *Infant Nutrition,* 2nd ed. Philadelphia, W.B. Saunders Co., 1974, pp. 360-370.

3.   Jelliffe DB and Jelliffe EFP: *Breast is best: Modern meanings.* NEJM 297:912-915, 1977.

4.   Applebaum RM: The obstetrician's approach to the breasts and breast feeding. J Reproductive Med 14:98-116, 1975.

5.   Resman BH, Blumenthal HP and Jusko WJ: Breast milk distribution of theobromine from chocolate. J. Pediatr 91:477-480, 1977.

6.   Yurchak AM and Jusko WJ: Theophylline secretion into breast milk. Pediatrics 57:518-520, 1976.

7.   Patton S and Keenan TW: The milk fat globule membrane. Biochim Biophys Acta 415:273-309, 1975.

8.   Vorherr H: *The Breast.* Academic Press, New York, 1974, pp.107-124.

9.   Kesaniemi YA: Ethanol and acetaldehyde in the milk and peripheral blood of lactating women after ethanol administration. Journal of Obstetrics and Gynaecology of the British Commonwealth 81:84-86, 1974.

10. Schanker LS: Passage of drugs across body membranes. Pharmacol Rev 14:501-530, 1962.

11. Rasmussen F: Excretion of drugs by milk. Chapter 20 in Brodie BB and Gilette JR (eds): *Handbook of Experimental Pharmacology* Vol 28. Concepts in Biochemical Pharmacology, Part 1. Springer-Verlag, New York, 1971, pp. 390-402.

12. Miller, GE, Banjee NC and Stowie CM Jr: Drug movement between bovine milk and plasma as affected by milk pH. J Dairy Sci 50:1395-1403, 1967.

13. Rasmussen F: Studies on the mammary excretion and absorption of drugs. Copenhagen: Fr. Martenson, 1966.

14. Rasmussen F: The mechanisms of drug secretion into milk. In: Galli G, Jacini G and Pecile A (eds). *Dietary Lipids and Postnatal Development.* Raven Press, New York, 1973, pp. 231-245.

15. Knowles, JA: Excretion of drugs in milk— A review. Pediatrics 66:1068-1082, 1965.

16. Savage RL: Drugs and Breast Milk Adverse Drug Reaction Bulletin (Pub. by Regional Postgraduate Institute for Medicine and Dentistry, Newcastle upon Tyne). No. 61, 212-225, 1976. Tyne). No. 61, 212-215, 1976.

17. Rivera-Calimlim L: Drugs in breast milk. Drug Therapy, pp. 59-63, December 1977.

18. Hervada AR, Feit E and Sagranes R: Drugs in breast milk. Perinatal Care 2:19-25, 1978.

19. O'Brien TE: Excretion of drugs in human milk. Amer J Hosp Pharm 31:844-854, 1974.

20. Catz CS and Giacola GP: Drugs and breast milk. Pediatr Clin N Amer 19:151-166, 1972.

21. Kwit NT and Hatcher RA: Excretion of drugs in milk. Amer J Dis Child 49:900-904, 1935.

22. Berlin DM: Antipyrine appearance and decay in human breast milk and saliva. Pharmacologist 20:219, 1978.

23. Yoshioka H, Cho K, Takimoto M, Maruyama S and Shimizu T: Transfer of cefazolin into human milk. J Pediatr 94:151-152, 1979.

24. Werthmann MW and Krees SV: Excretion of chlorothiazide in human breast milk. J Pediatr 81:781-783, 1972.

25. Cole AP and Hailey DM: Diazepam and active metabolite in breast milk and their transfer to the neonate. Arch Dis Child 50:741-742, 1975.

26. Loughnan PM: Digotoxin excretion in human breast milk. J Pediatr 92:1019-1020, 1978.

27. Berlin CM and Lee C: Isoniazid and acetylisoniazid disposition in human milk, saliva and plasma. Fed Proc 38:426,1979.

28. Schou M and Amdisen A: Lithium and pregnancy - III, Lithium ingestion by children breast fed by women on lithium treatment. Brit Med J 2:138, 1973.

29. Blinisk G and Inurrisi CE, Jerez E and Wallach RC: Methoadone assays in pregnant women and progeny. Amer J Obstet Gyn 121:617-621, 1975.

30. Ferguson BB, Wilson DJ and Schaffner W: Determination of nicotine concentrations in human milk. Am J Dis Child 130:837-839, 1976.

31. McKenzie SA, Selley JA and Agnew JE: Secretion of prednisolone into breast milk. Arch Dis Child 50:894-896, 1975.

32. Berlin CM, Debers L and Kaiser D: Prednisone and prednisolone in human milk after large oral dose of prednisone. Pharmacologist (in press).

33. Karlberg B, Lindberg D and Aberg H: Excretion of propranolol in human breast milk. Acta Pharmacol et toxicol 34:222-224, 1974.

34. Levy G: Salicylate pharmacokinetics in the human neonate, In Morselli PL, Garactini G and Sereni F (eds.), *Basic and Therapeutic Aspects of Perinatal Pharmacology,* Raven Press, 1975, pp 319-330.

35. Berlin CM and Yaffe SJ: Disposition of sulfasalazine (azulfidin) in human breast milk, plasma, and saliva. Pediatr Res (in press).

36. Dreisbach JA: Sulphone levels in breast milk of mothers on sulphone terapy. Lebrosy Review 23:101-106, 1952.

37. Wienick PH and Duncan JH: Cyclophosphamide in human milk. Lancet I:912, 1971.

38. Laug EP, Kunze FM and Prickett CS: Occurrence of DDT in human fat and milk. Arch Ind Hyg and Occ Med 3:245-246, 1951.

39. WHO/FAO. Pesticide Residues in Food. Technical Report Series No. 417, Geneva, 1969..

40. Brenik EM and Bjerk JE: Organochlorine compounds in Norwegian human fat and milk. Acta Pharmacol et toxicol 43:59-63, 1978.

41. Bakken, Arne F and Seip M: Insecticides in human breast milk. Acta Pediatr Scand 65: 535-539, 1976.

42. Siyali DS: Polychlorinated biphenyls, hexachlorobenzene and other organochlorine pesticides in human milk. Med J Australia 2:815-818, 1973.

43. Turistra LGMT: Organochlorine insecticide residues in human milk in one Leiden region. Netherlands Milk and Dairy Journal 25(1):24-32, 1971.

44. Holdrinet MVH, Braun HE, Frank R, Stopps GJ, Smout MS and McWade JW: Organochlorine residues in human adipose tissue and milk from Ontario residents 1969-74. Can J Public Health 68:74-80, 1977.

45. Quinby GE, Armstrong JF and Durham WF: DDT in human milk. Nature 207:726-728, 1965.

46. Kroger M: Insecticide residues in human milk. J Pediatr 80:401-405, 1972.

47. Brilliant LB, and Price H: Breast-milk monitoring to measure Michigan's contamination with polybrominated biphenyls. Lancet 2:643-646, 1978.

48. Vorherr H: *The Breast*. Academic Press, New York, 1974, pp 118-123.

49. Rasmussen F and Linzell JL: The Acetylation of sulphamalamide by mammary tissue of lactating goats. Biochem Pharmacol 16:918-919, 1967.

50. Dao TL: Studies on mechanism of carcinogenesis in the mammary gland. Prog Exp Tumur Res 11:235-261, 1969.

51. Bruder G, Fink A and Jarasch E-D: The B-Type cytochrome in endoplasmic reticulum of mammary gland epithelium and milk fat globule membranes consists of two components, cytochrome b_5 and cytochrome P-420. Esperimental Cell Research 117:207-217, 1978.

52. Liu DK, Kulick D and Williams GH: Ca^{2+}-stimulated ribonuclease. Biochem J 178:241-244, 1979.

53. Liu DK: Personal communication, 1979.

54. McCormick JJ, Larson LJ and Rich MA: RNase inhibition of reverse treanscriptase activity in human milk. Nature 251:737-740, 1974.

55. Scholm J, Spiegelman S and Moore DH: Detection of high molecular-weight RNA in particles from human milk. Science 175:542-544, 1972.

56. deSweet M, Lewis PJ: Excretion of anticoagulants in human milk. NEJM 297: 1471, 1977.

57. Whitelaw A, Butterfield A: High breast-milk sodium in cystic fibrosis. Lancet 2:1288, 1977.

58. Tobin RE and Schneider PB: Uptake of ^{67}Ga in the lactating breast and its persistence in milk: Case report. J Nuc Med 17:1055-1056, 1976.

59. Wyburn Jr: Human breast milk excretion of radionuclides following administration of radiopharmaceuticals. J Nuc Med 14:115-117, 1973.

60. Rumble WF, Aamodt RL, Jones AE, Henkin RI and Johnston GS: Accidental ingestion of Tc-99m in breast milk by a 10 week-old child. J Nuc Med 19:913-915, 1978.

Chapter 4

Breastfeeding—
Advantages and Issues

In this chapter we will first present the advantages of breastfeeding and then cover miscellaneous issues sometimes raised in discussions of breast- vs. bottle feeding.

NUTRITIONAL ADVANTAGES

Human milk is ideally adapted to the human infant. It has the nutrients, minerals and other substances needed for optimal human growth. The use of infant formulas has reached a high degree of sophistication and there now are many different types in use. Some are based on cow's milk protein; others use protein from other sources, such as soy. The fat in formulas may be cow's milk fat or vegetable fat. Various carbohydrates are used: lactose, sucrose, glucose, or corn starch with some formulas containing combinations. Specific vitamins and minerals may or may not be added. Some formulas come very close to breast milk in content and are called "humanized" by the manufacturer. However, even these formulas, as was shown by Table 2-1, are not exactly equivalent to breast milk.

Breast milk is the best digested and absorbed of all infant feeds. That stools of the breastfed infant are sweet smelling reflects the lack of undigested protein and fat present with formula feeds. They are loose and seedy as compared to the firmer, drier stools of the formula-fed baby. Constipation is rarely a problem. The breastfed baby who stools only once a week is not constipated; his stools are massive but always soft, while true constipation may be a real and frequent occurrence in the formula-fed infant.

The breastfed baby of a well-nourished mother receives adequate vitamins and minerals. He needs no supplements or other source of nutrition during the first four to six months of life, with the possible exception of vitamin D and fluoride.

Deficiency Syndromes

Various formulas have been responsible for deficiency syndromes when essential substances were inadvertently or unknowingly left out.

Acrodermatitis enteropathica, a rare genetic syndrome of diarrhea and dermatitis, is triggered by a zinc deficiency and occurs only in formula-fed infants. It is cured with breast-milk feeds or zinc supplements (1). Recently vitamin E deficiency was reported in premature infants when new formulas with higher levels of polyunsaturated fatty acids were fed. The increased requirement for vitamin E in the presence of high levels of polyunsaturated fats was unknown before this clinical deficiency was documented (2). Another example was the occurrence of seizures due to a pyridoxine deficiency in infants fed a specifically pyridoxine deficient formula (3).

Human milk may contain other substances as yet undescribed which are essential to normal growth. Creating a new formula will always entail the risk of inducing a new deficiency state.

Allergy

One of the commonest food allergies is cow's milk allergy. Soy formulas were developed as an alternative to formulas based on cow's milk. However, risk of allergy to soy protein may be as great as that to cow's milk protein (4,5).

It has been suggested that early exposure to allergens may cause allergic problems later in life to be more frequent and severe. This effect, possibly caused by the relative immaturity of the newborn's immune system, and hence his decreased ability to handle allergens such as foreign proteins, remains debated and as yet unproved (6).

Pediatricians and family practitioners have all seen and followed children with multiple formula intolerance. These infants often fail to thrive. They have recurrent episodes of diarrhea and sometimes vomiting. Multiple formula changes are attempted. At times the situation can become life-threatening. The best cure—breast milk—is often difficult to obtain. Relactation is possible, but difficult (see Chapter 13). In a child with a strong family history of allergies, breastfeeding has particularly clear advantages.

Obesity

Infantile obesity has become a significant problem in Western culture (7). Causes are multiple but often begin with the method of feeding. The breast-fed baby is ideally fed by demand—the baby's demand. The mother cannot tell how much he receives. There is a tendency for mothers who bottle feed to "finish the bottle." Bottle feeding gives the infant less control over the quantity of milk taken, and if the mother or grandmother feels more is better, there is a tendency to overfeed. Infants need sucking stimulation, most often beyond what is required to obtain enough calories. After 10-12 minutes the breastfed baby nurses on an essentially "empty" breast. He will always obtain some small amount of milk, but not the continued flow of 20 cal/oz as from a milk bottle. The bottle-fed baby who needs extra time sucking can be offered a pacifier.

The practice of over concentrating formula feeds by adding too little water during reconstitution is not an uncommon problem. These higher-concentration feeds have higher levels of electrolytes as well as more calories. This increase in electrolytes can cause increased thirst and therefore increased intake and can result in excessive weight gain. Hypernatremic dehydration also can occur in this setting, if extra water is not offered. Breast milk is a perfectly warmed, properly prepared milk which is ever ready. Its high free water content makes water supplements unnecessary.

Another factor preventing obesity in breastfed infants may be the variation in milk content during a feed. It is postulated that the rising fat content as milk is drained from the breast teaches the infant appetite control (8). A 3- or 4-month-old infant put to the breast nurses vigorously for 5-10 minutes. Most of the milk is emptied in that time and the fat content is then at its highest level. It is not unusual to observe the baby then begin to nurse less vigorously, or to stop nursing completely, as he apparently feels sated from the milk with the high-fat content. When he is then switched to the other breast, the baby begins to nurse vigorously again, slowing again as the breast is emptied. No infant food manufacturer has yet duplicated the variation of concentration of fat that occurs within each breastfeeding.

Coronary Protection

Western society is in the midst of an epidemic of atherosclerosis and coronary artery disease. Exact causes are unknown and are probably multiple, but a correlation between high serum cholesterol and heart disease does exist. Infant formulas have followed the general trend of the Western world to decrease saturated fat content in the diet and have begun using vegetable oils (which are mostly unsaturated fats and contain little cholesterol) in place of animal fats in infant formulas. The short-term effect of this is, as would be predicted, to lower serum cholesterol levels in bottle-fed infants compared to breastfed infants. Mean blood levels of 128 mg% for bottle fed vs. 146 mg% were found at 2-4 months in one study (9).

Of note is the fairly uniform and high concentration of cholesterol in human milk, despite alterations in maternal diet. Levels are estimated in recent studies to be between 12-24 mg% and are not dependent on changes in maternal diet (10,11,12).

A further observation has been made in rats. Adult rats that were maintained on artifically lowered cholesterol milks in early life have higher levels of cholesterol than those fed unaltered milk (13). Do young mammals need exposure to cholesterol in order to induce the enzymes necessary to maintain normal blood cholesterol levels in later life? The answer is unknown at present.

The high concentration of cholesterol in nervous tissue and the consistently high levels found in breast milk make the role of milk cholesterol during infancy—a time of rapid brain growth—an important question.

The long term effect of polyunsaturated vegetable fats or saturated cow's milk fat on brain growth and on coronary protection are unknown. To date there is no proof of a detrimental effect.

IMMUNOLOGICAL ADVANTAGES

Recently immunological properties of colostrum and breast milk have begun to be seriously investigated (14,15,16,17,18). Following is a list of immunological substances now known to be present in breast milk and colostrum: immunoglobulins, lysozyme, lactoferrin, complement, lactoperoxidase, macrophages, lymphocytes, interferon, "antistaphylococcal factor," and "bifidus factor."

It is an old clinical observation that breastfed infants are more resistant to infections, particularly gastro-intestinal infections, than are bottle-fed infants. In certain animal species (such as the cow, horse, and pig) it is known that failure of the newborn to suckle soon after birth results frequently in death from sepsis and diarrhea. In these species it has been documented that the colostrum contains immunoglobulins of all classes and that these are absorbed through the neonate's gut, despite the large size of the protein and later inability of such proteins to be absorbed (19). In these species the newborn is without benefit of maternal transfer of immunoglobulins in utero and is dependent on the first feeds of colostrum for immunological protection at birth. In humans, IgG is transferred across the placenta and offers considerable protection in the first weeks and first months of life. It has been assumed therefore that the immunoglobulins in human colostrum, which are mostly IgA, were of little clinical importance.

The relative resistance of the breastfed infant was assumed mostly to represent the bottle-fed infant's greater likelihood of receiving contaminated feeds. This could not, however, explain all. The occurrence of epidemics of Escherichia coli infection has been documented in nursery settings, where strict asepsis is practiced. Two such epidemics were documented to be unresponsive to isolation procedures, strict handwashing, closing of wards, and antibiotic therapy. The feeding of raw unprocessed breast milk was finally successful in ending both epidemics (20,21). It would appear then that breast milk must itself have protective properties. What are these properties?

Lactobacillus

It is well known that the stools of breastfed infants contain predominately lactobacilli while those of the formula fed contain mostly (like the adult) E. coli and other possible pathogenic gram negative organisms. Factors responsible for this are multiple. The presence of high concentrations of the breast-milk protein lactoferrin can be shown to be inhibitory to the growth of E. coli and, in combination with specific antibodies against E. coli, to be bacteriostatic (22). (Of note is the loss of this effect if the lactoferrin is saturated with iron, as might occur in vivo if iron supplements are given. However, the clinical significance of this observation is unclear at present.) The more acidic pH of the breastfed infant's stool, which reflects human milk's high lactose concentration and the more complete absorption of its fats and proteins, is also a factor. The acidity encourages growth of lactobacillus compared to that of E. coli and other gram negative organisms (23). The effect of formula supplements on the breastfed infant is to interfere with growth of lactobacillus, to elevate the pH of the stool and apparently then to decrease the protective effect of breastmilk feeds (24).

Lysozyme present in breast milk and documented in the stools of breastfed infants (but not in those of the formula fed) also inhibits the growth of E. coli in vitro and also may contribute to preferential growth of lactobacilli (25). The "bifidus factor," present in human milk and only minimally in cow's milk, is a growth factor described by György which is required by a particular species of lactobacillus, and is perhaps also a factor in the predominance of lactobacilli in the breastfed infant's gut (26).

Immunoglobulins

IgA is present in much higher concentrations in colostrum than in mature breast milk but both concentrations are much greater than in maternal plasma (27). The IgA of colostrum and milk now is known to be a secretory immunoglobulin. Unlike the monomeric serum IgA, it is a dimer consisting of two IgA particles connected by a secretory component. Secretory IgA from breast milk is, in virtro, resistant to acid and enzymic digestion (28). In vivo, specific IgA antibodies have been recovered from the stools of breastfed infants intact and in proportion to the levels present in the breast milk originally fed to the infant (28). Secretory IgA clearly survives passage through the alimentary tract. It appears to have an important role in the local immunity of the gut, an important site of local, and often subsequently, systemic infection during infancy (29).

Specific breast-milk antibodies correlate with maternal plasma antibodies and can be documented to multiple pathogens (14,30).

Role of Other Immunoglobulins and Cellular Immunity
It has generally been accepted that there is no absorption of immunoglobulins through the gut in the human neonate (as occurs in other species). Several recent studies however suggest the possible absorption of antibodies (31,32) as well as transfer of cellular-immunity to the breastfed infant in the first days of life (31). Relevance of these findings to the neonate's immune system needs further study.

Another possible immunological factor is the "anti-staphylococcal factor" described by György et al (33). Mice given a sublethal dose of staphylococci in combination with subcutaneous human milk were found to have protection against a subsequent lethal dose of staphylococci. The effect took several days to develop (perhaps demonstrating immunoglobulin induction?).

Cells Produce Immunological Substances
Colostrum and breast milk contain mononuclear cells, which are metabolically active, and of probable immunological significance (34). In vitro milk macrophages can be shown to produce lysozyme, C3, C4, and possibly lactoferrin (35). The lymphocytes (10% of mononuclear cells present) have been characterized as approximately ½ B and ½ T cells, which in vitro can be shown to produce secretory IgA, interferon, migration inhibition factor, and possibly lymphokines (35,36,37,38). It is unclear what role these cells have in the immunological protection of the newborn and infant, but it has been shown that induction and secretion of specific immunoglobulins into colostrum occurs in response to new organisms introduced into the maternal gut (39). This observation suggests a transfer of immunological information between maternal gut (Peyer's patch) lymphocytes and colostral and breast-milk lymphocytes. This transfer of immunological information within the mother from the mesenteric nodes of her gut to the breast probably is accomplished by migration of lymphocytes. It appears that lymphocytes from the gut, capable of transformation into plasmablasts, carry the information and travel to the breast, with production and secretion of specifically induced secretory IgA into colostrum (and breast milk).

Necrotizing Enterocolitis (NEC)
Another indication of the importance of the macrophages and lymphocytes in breast milk is the observation in rats of protection from NEC, in an experimental model of the disease, by maternal milk (40). The protective effect can be strongly related to the living cells in the maternal milk (41).

Epidemiology

What does all this mean to well-cared-for Western infants? Recent epidemiological studies comparing breastfed with formula-fed infants are hard to evaluate. Study numbers tend to be small. One recent study indicated definite increased protection in breastfed infants with significantly fewer illnesses and serious illnesses occuring during infancy (42). Decreased incidence of gastrointestinal disease is most clearly documented in several studies (43,44,45). Perhaps the most impressive study, however, is that of Grulee et al., published in 1934 (46). Between 1924 and 1929, he studied over 20,000 infants who attended Infant Welfare Society clinics in Chicago. Medical supervision was readily available and children were seen at least monthly by a visiting nurse. Breastfeeding was encouraged: 48.5% were entirely breastfed, 43% were partially breastfed, and 8.5% were formula-fed. Most striking were the mortality data: 66.1% of the deaths occurred in the formula-fed group, although they represented only 8.5% of the total population. Six and seven-tenths percent of the deaths which occurred were in the totally breastfed group, and 27.2% in the partly breastfed. This distribution was consistent for deaths from GI infections and from respiratory infections. About 1/3 of the breastfed group developed an infection during the first 9 months, 2/3 of the formula fed, and 1/2 of the supplemented group. This morbidity reflected mostly GI infections; 16% of the formula-fed developing GI infections compared to only 5% of the breastfed. (Some of this increased morbidity may have reflected poor sterilization techniques and inadequate refrigeration, which is a less frequent occurrence today.)

ECONOMY

The question of relative costs of breastfeeding vs. bottle feeding is an important one. The cost of breastfeeding depends on the mother's diet. Breastfeeding can be as cheap or as expensive as the mother's diet. It is a question of whether the extra calories are obtained from peanut butter or from filet mignon. Six hundred to eight hundred Cal/day is estimated to be the energy cost of lactation per day, some of which can be obtained initially from extra weight put on during pregnancy. Depending on the types of foods used, from "thrifty" to "liberal," costs were estimated by one author in 1976 to range from $3 to $5/week, assuming 800 ml. of breast milk produced per day as an approximate maximal output (47). The range of costs for formula per week (28 oz/day) are $4.67 (powder) to $4.73 (cans) to $20.00 in ready-to-serve nursette bottles. Additional money would be required to cover the cost of bottles, nipples and energy for heating water, sterilizing, etc.

The natural resources and energy used in making, processing, bottling and distributing infant formula are another consideration. Even in the wealthy Western world, the question of priorities of energy use may one day be an argument for breastfeeding. The 90% estimated energy efficiency of breast-milk production cannot be matched by any other baby food manufacturing and delivery process.

CONVENIENCE

The first weeks after the birth of a baby are transitional ones, regardless of the feeding technique. Parents are learning new roles and responsibilities. The baby is learning about his new environment. At times, the continuous attention needed by a newborn may seem to be overwhelming to parents. The frequency of feedings required by most nursing babies is seen as an added inconvenience. However, by two months, when baby begins to sleep a little longer at night and is more alert by day, the rewards of nursing begin to make even very difficult first weeks seem worthwhile to most breast-feeding couples. The social smile of the 2-month old is powerful reinforcement to mothering (and fathering).

The breastfed baby is portable; he travels easily, requiring mostly his mother. Nutrition and comfort are ever-ready.

To other mothers, however, bottle feeding is a more convenient choice. It allows them more freedom from the very beginning. For the mother who plans to return to work soon after delivery, convenience cannot be cited as an advantage of breastfeeding. Yet many women still choose to nurse, believing the inconvenience is worth the other benefits of a nursing relationship. Working and nursing are discussed in Chapter 11.

PSYCHOLOGICAL ADVANTAGES

Psychological advantages of breastfeeding are more difficult to document clinically than immunological or nutritional advantages, but they also are of significance. An examination of breastfeeding would be incomplete without considering its psychological aspects.

One cannot examine the breastfeeding literature without noting that most of the material that describes psychological aspects of breastfeeding has been written by women who have nursed their own children. The psychological aspects of lactation are important especially in the minds of those with personal experience (48,49,50,51,52,53).

In attempts to encourage pregnant women to breastfeed their babies, the physical advantages of breast milk to the infant, or the advantages of economy or convenience to the mother, often are cited. Yet the psychological factors—the emotions, the enjoyment by both the mother and infant in the feeding situation—may be more significant factors in the minds of women who actually breastfeed. Perhaps a more effective campaign to convince pregnant women of the advantages of breastfeeding would cite the

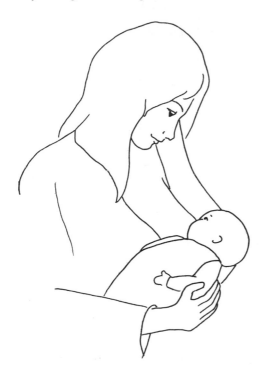

Figure 4-1. *En face* nursing.

psychological advantages. Unlike other advantages, which mainly are for either the infant (e.g., immunological factors), or mainly for the mother (e.g., economy), the psychological advantages apply to the nursing couple as a synchronous unit.

The human infant needs adequate nutrition, warmth, love, environmental stimulation and rest. Unlike most other mammalian newborns, the human neonate is immobile and completely dependent for many months after birth. The importance of consistent mothering during these early months is well recognized. The human infant needs to be loved and cuddled; he needs consistent reliable care. An important part of learning to form close human attachments, to love, is in being loved (54).

All the above needs of the newborn and young infant are met by breast-feeding. Obviously these needs can be met in other ways, but breastfeeding is uniquely suited to meeting all the infants' needs in one act. As the modern world becomes more complex and technological, this simple act of love between two human beings seems all the more precious.

The interactions between mother and child are, in a sense, a fail-safe system to ensure the proximity of mother and child. Breastfeeding provides a synchronous giving and taking, a reciprocal interaction: simultaneously giving emotional and physical pleasure to both mother and child.

It may be incorrect to attempt to separate psychological factors from physiological ones (55). There is no doubt that humans act "motherly" without the high prolactin levels that are associated with lactation, but the higher prolactin levels may be an advantage to the new mother. It has been hypothesized that prolactin may enhance a mother's attachment to her child. The release of oxytocin during suckling is associated with feelings of well being and relaxation in many women, feelings that are reported to resemble those following orgasm. Most women describe the time spent nursing an infant as peaceful and pleasurable; sometimes, these periods are highlights in an otherwise hectic day. The successfully nursing mother needs no reminding to enjoy relaxed and leisurely feedings.

Lactation is one of woman's sexual functions, a culmination of intercourse, pregnancy and childbirth. "For a *baby* who cannot be breastfed, there is a substitute food, however imperfect. For the *mother* who cannot breastfeed, there is no real substitute" (56).

The successfully breastfeeding mother, who nurses to give comfort as well as to give nutrition, evolves a different set of responses to her child than the bottle-feeding mother or the breastfeeding mother who nurses only to allay hunger. In Western culture, it is often believed that during the newborn period, hunger is the main discomfort and is the main cause for crying. But sometimes babies cry from an unknown cause. The mother who sees breastfeeding as comfort does not hesitate to offer the breast at these times.

This difference in approach to the baby becomes more marked as the baby gets older. The 4-month-old whose DPT shot is hurting him, the 6-month-old who is lonely, and the 9-month-old who has tried to stand and has bumped his head, may all be comforted by nursing.

Without an understanding of these psychological aspects of normal lactation (synchronous mother-infant unit, nursing as comfort, feedings on demand), breastfeeding is unlikely to continue past the early days or weeks, and thus the other advantages of breastfeeding are also partially lost.

NURSING-BOTTLE CARIES

Children and older infants who are allowed to sleep with a bottle of formula or other sweetened drink and who suck on the bottle through the night are at risk for extensive tooth decay. The teeth most directly bathed in the formula or beverage are most usually involved (front upper teeth). Breastfed infants, even those who nurse intermittently through the night, are not so affected.

POSITIONAL OTITIS MEDIA AND BOTTLE PROPPING

An increased incidence of otitis media has been noted in bottle-fed babies who are frequently fed in the horizontal position compared with bottle-fed infants never fed in that position (57). Propping bottles is not uncommon and even occurs on busy pediatric wards. This practice is unfortunate.

The breastfed infant is assured the stimulation of being held and cuddled during feedings and also has the advantage of increased immunological protection. "Feeding times are the most joyous moments of the young infant's life. The close face-to-face association of mother and infant during nursing (or bottle feeding when baby is held and cuddled) not only serves to link in the baby's mind this happiness with his mother but may form the basis for the importance of mealtime to the family unit in later life." (58)

SUDDEN INFANT DEATH SYNDROME (SIDS)(59)

At present there is no clear relation between method of feeding and SIDS (60), although various factors which might be related to a possible protective effect of breastfeeding have been noted and include the following: [1] many SIDS victims have some mild infectious illness at time of death, [2] electrolyte abnormalities or dehydration are suggested by elevated electrolyte concentrations found in the vitreous humor in some cases, [3] some unproven theories involve an allergic pathogenesis involving foreign milk protein (61). Overlying, once believed to be a common factor, is not usually a possible cause, since most victims die alone.

BREAST CANCER

Epidemiological evidence from a large international study showed no relation between nursing and breast cancer: no protection, no increased risk. However, the incidence of breast cancer in countries where breastfeeding is prevalent is lower (62,63). Past claims of viral particles in human milk of women with strong family histories of breast cancer, similar to particles known to transmit mice mammary carcinoma (64), have not been substantiated (65,66).

Observation of an increased risk of breast cancer in the unsuckled breast of women of Hong Kong who traditionally use only one side to nurse with, is interesting. Further research is indicated (67).

Breast cancer publicity and breast self-examination have made women very concerned about any lump in the breast. Lumps and a lumpiness are quite common in the lactating breast, especially in the early weeks. A lump may be the result of a plugged duct or a swollen area of localized engorgement. It may be a harmless cyst, filled with milk. A lump that first appears during lactation is likely to be related to nursing. Women are sometimes quite frightened, feeling certain that any new lump is a sign of cancer. In most cases, differentiation is not difficult, as a lump that has appeared during lactation can usually be observed to change in size and shape and may resolve.

A lactating woman whose lump has not changed at all in size or position should be seen by a gynecologist familiar with the lactating breast. Breast cancer, although more rare than plugged ducts or engorgement, has been diagnosed in the lactating breast.

THE WOMEN'S LIBERATION MOVEMENT

Margaret Mead described the women's liberation movement as having two extreme factions, the group seeking to destroy all remnants of differences between male and female, and those who wish to allow women to express more fully their femininity, to remove constraints placed on modern woman by Western culture, and to allow the woman who bears children to nurture her children fully (52). For this later group breastfeeding is an obvious source of pleasure and satisfaction which every woman has the right to enjoy.

It is paradoxical that the bottle feeding that was intended to liberate mothers also downgraded their importance, while the breast feeding that was thought to enslave them makes it perfectly clear to everyone, especially the mother, that she is of unique and irreplaceable value (68).

The working mother has special needs, but increasingly women are combining a return to work with successful breastfeeding. (See Chapter 11.)

References

1. Jelliffe, DB and Jelliffe, EFP: *Human Milk In the Modern World.* Oxford: Oxford Press, 1978.

2. Oski, FA and Barness, LA: Vitamin E deficiency: previously unrecognized cause of hemolytic anemia in the premature infant. J.Pediatr. 70:211, 1967.

3. Courson, OB: Convulsive seizures in infants with pyridoxine deficient diets. JAMA 154: 406, 1954.

4. Halpern, et al.: Development of childhood allergy in infants fed breast, soy or cow milk. J. Allergy Clin. Immunol. 51: 139, 1973.

5. Eastman, FJ, et al.: Antigenicity of infant formulas: role of immature intestine on protein permeability. J. Pediatr. 93: 561, 1978.

6. Taylor, B et al.: Transient IgA deficiency and pathogenesis of infantile atopy. Lancet 2:111, 1973.

7. Jelliffe, S and Jelliffe, EFD: Fat babies—prevalence, perils and prevention. J. of Trop. Pediatr. & Environmental Child Health 124, 1975.

8. Hall, B. Changing composition of human milk and early development of an appetite control. Lancet 1: 179, 1975.

9. Friedman, G, Goldberg, SJ: Concurrent and subsequent serum cholesterol of breast and formula fed infants. Am. J. Clin. Nutr. 28:42, 1975.

10. Guthrie, et al.: Fatty acid composition of human milk. J. Pediatr. 90:39, 1977.

11. Mellios, MJ et al.: Effects of varying maternal dietary cholesterol and phytosterol in lactating women and their infants. Amer. J. Clin. Nutr. 31: 1347, 1978.

12. Potter, JM et al.: The effects of dietary fatty acids and cholesterol on the milk lipids of lactating women. Am. J. Clin. Nutr. 29: 54, 1976.

13. Reiser, R, Sidelman, Z: Control of serum cholesterol homeostasis by cholesterol in the milk of the suckling rat. J. Nutr. 102: 1009, 1972.

14. Goldman, AS and Smith, CW: Host resistance factors in human milk. J. Pediatr. 82: 1082m 1973,

15. Hanson, LA and Winberg, J: and defence against infection in the newborn. Arch. Dis. Child 47: 845, 1972.

16. Gerrard,JW:Breastfeeding: second thoughts, Pediatr. 54: 757, 1974.

17. Mata, LJ and Wyatt, RG: Host resistance to infection. Am. J. Clin. Nutr. 24: 976, 1971.

18. Winberg, J and Wessner, G: Does breast milk protect against septicaemia in the newborn. Lancet 1: 1091, 1971.

19. Kon, SK and Cowie, AK: *The Mammary gland and Its Secretion.* New York: Academic Press, 1961.

20. Surusky-Grass, S: Pathogenic strains of E. Coli among prematures and use of human milk in controlling outbreak of diarrhea. Ann. Pediatr. 190:109, 1958.

21. Largua, AM et al.: Fresh human colostrum for the prevention of E. Coli diarrhea—a clinical experience. J. Trop. Pediatr. 23: 289, 1977.

22. Bullen, JJ et al.: Iron-binding proteins in milk and resistance to E. coli infections in infants. Br. Med. J.L: 69, 1972.

23. Bullen, CL and Tearle, PV: Bifidobacteria in the intestinal tract of infants: an in-vitro study. J. Med. Microbiol. 9: 335, 1976.

24. Bullen, CL et al.: The effect of "humanized" milks and supplemented breastfeeding on the faeces flora of infants. J. Med. Microbiol. 10: 403, 1977.

25. Rosenthal, L and Lieberman, H: The role of lysozyme in the development of the intestinal flora of the new-born infant. Infed. Dis. 48: 226, 1931.

26. György, P: Biochemical aspects in The Uniqueness of Human milk. Am. J. of Clin. Nutr. 24:970, 1971.

27. Ste-Marie, MT et al.: Radioimmunologic measurements of naturally occurring antibodies, III. antibodies reactive with E. coli or bacteroides fragilis in breast fluids and sera of mothers and new born infants. Pediatr. Res. 8:815, 1974.

28. Kenny, JF et al.: Bacterial and viral coproantibodies in breastfed infants. Pediatr. 39: 202, 1967.

29. Galant, SP: Biological and clinical significance of the gut as a barrier to penetration of macromolecules. Clin. Pediatr. 15: 731, 1976.

30. Michael, JG et al.: The antimicrobial activity of human colostral antibody in the newborn. J. Infect. Dis. 124: 445, 1971.

31. Ogra, SS et al.: Immunologic aspects of colostrum and milk. III. fate and absorption of cellular and solunle components in the gastrointestinal tract of the newborn. J. Immunol. 119: 245, 1977.

32. Iyengar I and Selvaraj, RJ: Intestinal absorption of immunoglobulins by newborn infants. Arch. Dis. Child 47: 411, 1972.

33. György, P et al: Protective effects of human milk in experimental staphlococcus infection. Science 137: 338, 1962.

34. Lawton, JWM and Shortbridge, KF: Protective factors in human breast milk and colostrum. Lancet 1: 254, 1977.

35. Pitt, J: Breast milk leukocytes. Pediatrics 58: 769, 1976.

36. Smith, CW and Goldman, AS: The cells of human colostrum. I. In vitro studies of morphology and functions. Pediatr. Res. 2: 103, 1968.

37. Murillo, GJ and Goldman, AS: The cells of human colostrum. II. synthesis of IgA and BIC. Pediatr. Res. 4: 71, 1970.

38. Goldman, AS: Immunological aspects of breastfeeding, Sixth Annual Seminar on Breastfeeding for Physicians (sponsored by La Leche League International). Oct. 20, 1978.

39. Goldblum, RM et al.: Antibody-forming cells in human colostrum after oral immunization. Nature 257: 797, 1975.

40. Barlow B et al.: An experimental study of acute neonatal enterocolitis: the importance of breast milk. J. Pediatr. Sug. 9: 587, 1974.

41. Pitt, J et al.: Macrophages and the protective action of breast milk in necrotizing enterocolitis. Ped. Res. 8: 384, 1974.

42. Cunningham, AS: Morbidity in Breastfed and artificially fed infants. J. Pediatr. 90: 726, 1977.

43. Robinson, M: Infant morbidity and mortality. Lancet 1: 768, 1951.

44. Stewart, A and Westropp, C: Breast-feeding in the Oxford child health survey. Part II. Comparison of bottle-fed and breast-fed babies. Brit. Med. J. 2: 305, 1953.

45. Larsen, SA and Homer, DR: Relation of breast versus bottle feeding to hospitalization for gastroenteritis in a middle-class U.S. population. J. Pediatr. 92: 417, 1978.

46. Grulee, CG et al.: Breast and artificial feeding. JAMA 103: 735, 1934.

47. Lamm, E et al.: Economy in the feeding of infants. Pediatr. Clin. N.A. 24:71, 1977.

48. Weichert, C: Breastfeeding, first thoughts. Pediatrics 56: 987, 1975.

49. Newton, N: Psychological aspects of lactation. New Engl. J. Med. 277: 1479, 1967.

50. Gunther, M: The new mother's view of herself. CIBA Foundation Symposium 45 : 152, 1976.

51. Helsing, E: Lactation education; the learning of the 'obvious'. CIBA Foundation 45: 224, 1976.

52. Raphael, D: *The Tender Gift: Breastfeeding*. Englewood Cliffs, New Jersey: Prentice Hall, 1973.

53. Pryor, K: *Nursing Your Baby*. New York: Pocket Book Division of Simon and Schuster, 1973

54. Fraiberg, S: *In Defence of Mothering, Every Child's Birthright*. Basic Books, 1977.

55. Klaus, M and Kennel, J: *Maternal-Infant Bonding*. St. Louis: The C.V. Mosby Company, 1976.

56. Lloyd, JK: Chairman's introduction. CIBA Foundation Symposium 45:1, 1976.

57. Beauregard, WG: Positional otitis media. J. Pediatr. 70:294, 1971.

58. Nelson, JD: Prop the baby, not the bottle. J. Pediatr. 79:348, 1971.

59. Hasselmeyer, EG: The sudden infant death syndrome. in *Pediatrics*, Rudolph, AM, ed. New York: Appleton-Century, Crofts, 1977, p. 831.

60. Carpenter, E: Identification and follow-up of infants with sudden infant death syndrome. Nature 250:729, 1974.

61. Mathews, IS and Soothill: Hypersensitivity to milk and sudden infant death syndrome. Lancet 2:893, 1970.

62. MacMahon, B et al.: Lactation and cancer of the breast, a summary of an international study. Bulletin WHO 42:185, 1970.

63. Lowe, CR and MacMahon, B: Breast cancer and reproductive history of women in South Wales. Lancet 1:153, 1970.

64. Schlom, J and Splegleman, S: Detection of high molecular weight RNA in particles from human milk. Science 175:542, 1972.

65. Morgan et al.: Breastfeeding, family history, and breast disease. Amer. J. Epidemiol. 99:117, 1974.

66. Miller, R and Fraumenti, J: Does breast-feeding increase the child's risk of breast cancer? Pediatrics 49:645, 1972.

67. Ing, R et al.: Unilateral breast-feeding and breast cancer. Lancet 2:124, 1977.

68. Glickman, BM and Springer, BNB: *Who Cares for the Baby?* New York: Schocken Books, 1978.

Chapter 5

Pregnancy

THE DECISION TO BREASTFEED

At a prenatal visit during the second trimester, it is appropriate to ask the expectant mother how she is planning to feed her baby. Asking the question in this manner allows for an open discussion to follow. This discussion can be initiated by the physician or midwife who is giving prenatal care, or by a nurse, or another health professional in the physician's office or clinic.

The middle trimester is a good time to initiate this discussion. By this time the mother has felt the baby moving, she is feeling better and is probably receptive to new information.

For the woman who has made up her mind to bottle feed, and to whom breastfeeding is unappealing, no further discussion of breastfeeding may be appropriate although further discussion may uncover misconceptions that can be discussed. It has been suggested that many women are aware of the merits of breastfeeding and that, of these, those who have made a firm decision to bottle feed will hardly be convinced by logical arguments (1).

Some women will assume that they will bottle feed because they have never seen a woman breastfeeding. A discussion during the second trimester allows expectant parents who are undecided or who are first considering the possibility time to discuss the decision, to ask questions, and possibly to read a book on breastfeeding (such as Pryor's *Nursing Your Baby,* or Raphael's *The Tender Gift*). It is appropriate to discuss the advantages of breastfeeding for the infant and the advantages for the mother both with women who are undecided and with those who are already interested in breastfeeding. Information on all feeding methods should be given to all expectant parents. Once a parental decision has been made, this decision should be firmly supported.

The breastfeeding discussion should center on the advantages that are most meaningful to the pregnant woman. Perhaps the most compelling one is that breastfeeding can be a beautiful, emotionally gratifying experience, that it is a physically pleasurable part of motherhood.

As indicated in the earlier chapters, for the baby, breast milk is optimal nutrition: it is the best food for the young infant; it avoids the possibility of food allergy—which is of particular importance when there is a family history of allergic diseases; and breastfed babies have fewer infections and tend to be healthier.

Ideally, the expectant father is included in the discussion. This is a good time to discuss prenatal classes with both expectant parents.

Suggestions for further reading can be given (see Appendix A). The expectant mother can be told about local breastfeeding support groups.

A woman who has reached a decision in favor of breast-or bottle feeding should be supported in her decision. Not infrequently women in the late months of pregnancy state that they intend to breastfeed for only a limited time period, say six weeks or three months. This desire to control the duration of the coming experience is understandable in a woman whose current situation—pregnancy—seems to be endless. In fact many of these women continue to nurse longer, but their statement of intent should be supported.

PRENATAL CLASSES

Increasingly, expectant parents are attending classes about childbirth which encourage involvement of fathers during labor and delivery. These classes may also offer information about breastfeeding, and afford an ideal opportunity to discuss the advantages of breastfeeding with both parents. Ideally, childbirth classes help make labor and delivery less fearful. The mother who is able to relax during labor and delivery can be expected to need less analgesia and/or anaesthesia (2). The risks and benefits of maternal medications to mother and newborn also can be discussed with the pregnant woman along with an explanation of the course of normal childbirth.

NIPPLE PREPARATION

At the first prenatal visit it is customary to examine the expectant woman's breasts and nipples. "Poorly protractile" (flat or inverted) nipples can be identified and noted. Occasionally there is some doubt about the nipple type (see Fig. 5-1). An inverted nipple can be identified by using what has been called the "pinch test."

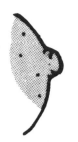 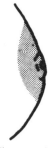 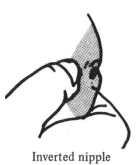

Common nipple   Flat nipple   Inverted nipple

Figure 5-1. Nipple types.

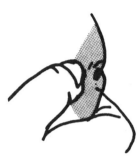

The Pinch Test

Using the thumb and forefinger, gently pinch the nipple at its base. If the nipple retracts or shrinks back, it is considered to be inverted.

Most often there is spontaneous improvement in non-protractile nipples during the nine months of gestation; however, a certain percentage of women with inverted nipples at the first prenatal visit will continue to have some degree of inversion or poorly protractile nipples at term; these conditions are estimated to persist in 5%-20% of the individuals (3).

Inverted nipples are a cause of pain, discomfort, and lactation failure and often are not improved by the suckling of the baby alone, contrary to common opinion. Prenatal nipple preparation, however, frequently can alleviate the problem prior to delivery and avoid this significant cause of lactation difficulty. Nipple preparation is definitely recommended for any woman with flat or inverted nipples who wants to breastfeed.

Each woman whose nipples were noted to be flat or inverted in early pregnancy should be re-examined at the beginning of the third trimester. If one or both nipples are still poorly protractile, she can be instructed in the Hoffman technique and in the use of the milk cup during the weeks remaining prior to delivery. The nipple exercise can be added later as an option.

The Hoffman Technique (4)

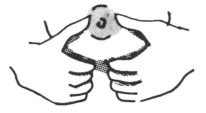

Place the thumbs opposite each other on either side of the nipple. Gently draw the thumbs away from the nipple. Then place the thumbs above and below the nipple and repeat. This should be done twice a day for a few minutes.

Figure 5-2. The Hoffman technique.

The Milk Cup

The milk cup works by applying steady, gentle pressure on the areola; it forces the nipple to extend forward. (It is also called a "breast shield." The original model was the Woolwich Shield.) (see Fig. 5-3.)

Instructions in the use of a milk cup (5)

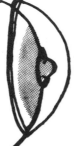

Begin by wearing the cup under the bra for short periods of time and gradually work up to 8 to 10 hours/ day. Be sure to allow air to circulate on the skin by removing the cup for short periods, or by wearing only the base part. Wearing the cup is painless.

Figure 5-3. A milk cup.

The Nipple Exercise

The nipple exercise is also referred to as "nipple rolling". It can be done by women with normal or flat nipples. The woman with inverted nipples should first do the Hoffman technique and wear a milk cup; after the woman is able to grasp her nipple, the nipple exercise may also be added to the routine (see Fig. 5-4).

Nipple exercise instructions

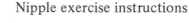

Support the breast with one hand and use the other hand for the exercise. Pull the nipple gently but firmly outward and roll the nipple between the thumb and finger. Then move the thumb and finger to another location at the base of the nipple and repeat.

Figure 5-4. The nipple exercise.

By the third trimester, most women have normally protractile nipples; for them, no formal nipple preparation is required. Some women are offended by the idea of being required to do specific nipple preparation routines or find it "too much trouble" (6). They simply may be advised to avoid using soap or other drying agents (e.g. alcohol) on the nipples during pregnancy and postpartum.

Other women, however, want to "do something" concrete to prepare for breastfeeding, perhaps largely for psychological reasons. For these women, some form of nipple preparation may be appropriate. Many different routines have been suggested, some of uncertain value, there being debate as to whether nipple preparation is effective at all. It is important to clarify in what specific respect a given routine is hoped to be effective.

One goal of nipple preparation is for the woman to become accustomed to handling her own breasts. There do not seem to be any studies on this point but it would seem that women who handle their breasts during pregnancy would feel more comfortable handling their breasts postpartum.

Another major goal of nipple preparation is to draw the nipples out so that they will be easier for the baby to grasp. Experience with the milk cup and with the Hoffman technique has shown repeatedly that these two measures are effective in increasing nipple protractility.

Yet another major goal of prenatal nipple preparation is freedom from soreness postpartum; sore nipples occur in many women in Western cultures, where nipples always are covered and therefore not toughened.

In a study conducted to test the effectiveness of traditional methods of nipple preparation in preventing soreness (7), the following methods were evaluated: nipple rolling for a period of 3-6 weeks, applying Masse cream for 3-6 weeks, and hand expressing colostrum for 3-6 weeks. In order to test whether nipple preparation prevented postnatal nipple pain and trauma, the women were instructed to prepare one breast only, twice daily for the 3-6 week period. (Women with non-protractile nipples, for whom nipple preparation is clearly indicated, were not studied). No significant difference was found between the prepared and unprepared breasts. It was concluded that the three routines were not effective in preventing soreness. No difference in soreness was found between redheaded women and other women (as often is claimed).

Hand expressing colostrum has been a commonly recommended prenatal routine. The woman who hand expresses colostrum is likely to be reassured to see that her breasts are producing colostrum, and there is the benefit that she will know how to hand express after delivery (However, learning how to do so postpartum is easy with appropriate teaching.)

The practice of routinely hand expressing colostrum may not however be advisable, and it is now less recommended than in the past (8). There is no evidence that it prevents soreness (7). With the exception of the reassurance, then, that colostrum exists, there is no evidence that the practice accomplishes anything that cannot be accomplished in other ways. Freedom from engorgement postpartum is best accomplished by early frequent nursings. Increased protractility is best accomplished by the Hoffman technique and the use of a milk cup.

In addition, there may be disadvantages to routinely hand expressing colostrum during pregnancy:

1. Possible opening of the ducts to hospital-borne infection (9).
2. Possible wasting of valuable colostrum (10) (No data exist on quantity of colostrum present or the effect of prenatal removal of some.)
3. Possible triggering of premature labor in a few susceptible women; pumping the breasts has been used successfully as a method of inducing labor (11).

Since there is no convincing argument to support the routine hand expression of colostrum, and since there may be disadvantages, other types of nipple preparation may be better recommended to women who want to prepare their breasts.

Another questionable, but frequently suggested, prenatal routine is rubbing the nipples with a towel in the hope that the friction of the rubbing will "toughen" the nipple/areola skin. After a few weeks of nursing, the nipple skin becomes toughened and a woman who has been nursing for some time may have a small callous on her nipple/areola skin, which can be seen on the underside of the nipple. However, it is uncertain that the friction from rubbing with a towel will cause similar toughening.

The persistence of personal testimonials and opinions to the effectiveness of various nipple preparation techniques in preventing postpartum problems may reflect other factors. Women who receive nipple preparation advice are probably less likely to become sore or engorged, as has often been claimed, but the reasons for this may not be the result of nipple preparation. The lay or medical advisor who is interested enough in breastfeeding to give nipple preparation advice is very likely to be interested enough to also give postpartum advice. Since women are usually still in contact with the same advisor after childbirth, they may therefore be helped to avoid nursing indiscretions (nursing on a four-hour schedule, using soap on the nipples, wearing plastic-lined bra pads, etc.) Nursing indiscretions *do* correlate with soreness and engorgement. Thus women may be avoiding or minimizing such problems mainly because they are in continuing contact with an interested advisor, rather than because of the efficacy of a particular nipple preparation routine. (see Chapter 8)

Other activities in a woman's life may be overlooked as factors in nipple preparation. Sexual activity involving the breast does help to increase nipple protractility and may toughen the skin. Similarly, exposure to light and air and avoidance of soap are unconscious, yet effective, nipple-preparation activities for many women.

A woman who wants to prepare her nipples can be advised to do the nipple exercise (see the instructions earlier in this chapter).

QUESTIONS ASKED BY PREGNANT WOMEN

Many young women have some reservations or questions about breastfeeding that can be answered during prenatal visits. Commonly asked questions are listed below, along with possible responses.

1. My breasts are small. Will I have enough milk for a baby?

Yes. Breast size correlates most closely with fat, not with amount of glandular tissue present. There is no correlation between breast size and milk supply.

2. If I breastfeed will I lose my figure? Will my breasts sag?

Changes in breast size after nursing are believed to reflect effects of pregnancy. In fact, optimally, extra weight is gained during pregnancy; and nursing helps the woman to lose that weight. After the milk comes in postpartum, the nursing mother will have fuller, larger breasts than if she had bottle fed and may need larger blouses and sweaters during the first weeks and months of lactation. These changes slowly reverse during the months postpartum, even during continued nursing. Most women find themselves back to pre-pregnancy size by nine months postpartum.

3. How do I know I'll have enough milk? My sister (my mother) didn't.

A woman will have enough milk if she nurses enough, that is, approximately every 2-2½-3 hours. She won't have enough milk if she doesn't. Women who say that their milk just dried up did not understand that milk production works by supply and demand, that is, "the more you nurse, the more milk you will have." Your sister (or mother) may have been trying to nurse according to the clock, or maybe tried to stave off feedings with bottles or solid food. Any woman will keep making milk as long as she nurses frequently.

4. Will my man feel left out if I breastfeed?

Fathers sometimes do feel left out after the mother and new baby come home from the hospital; this can happen because the mother is so busy with the new baby, regardless of whether or not she is breastfeeding. Unfortunately, fathers of breastfed babies sometimes worry that the only job left for them is changing diapers. This is not true. Babies have more needs than food and clean pants. They need to be held, cuddled, talked to, bathed, and loved—all things that fathers can learn to do well. While mothers naturally seem to spend more time in physical care, fathers seem naturally to spend more time in playing or talking to the baby.

The father of a breastfed baby in a predominantly bottle-feeding culture can play an additional role. He can be a source of support and reassurance to his wife when she has doubts. A father who is supportive of breastfeeding can be much more helpful than female relatives who are familiar only with bottle feeding, especially if he is interested and wants to have his baby breastfed.

5. My man thinks breastfeeding is dirty and animalistic.

How do you feel about breastfeeding? If you and your man feel very differently about this, you need to discuss it and come to some sort of understanding. Obviously you need to make a decision. Should you try to nurse when you have a disapproving man? It will not be easy. Such feelings are often not easily changed. A publication that is widely "consulted" on the subject of women's breasts (*Playboy*) recommended in one such case that professional help be sought for the man (12).

6. Will I be tied down if I decide to breastfeed?

Breastfed babies are very portable; you can grab a few diapers and go. Or you can leave your baby at home with a sitter and a bottle. It is up to you. If you want to be sure that your baby will take a bottle, it is important to get him used to taking a bottle. You can start offering a bottle a couple of times a week, or even once a day, if you want to; it's better to wait to begin introducing the bottle until after your baby has learned to nurse, when he is approximately two weeks old.

The fear of being tied down is a very common one, but it may be an exaggerated one. Most new mothers end up doing most of the feedings in the early weeks, regardless of whether they are breast-or bottle feeding. A bottle-feeding mother can go out and miss a feeding as long as she can find someone to give her baby the bottle. But then again, so can a breastfeeding mother, so long as she sees to it that her baby is used to taking a bottle.

Whether or not you want your nursing baby to have bottles is up to you.

7. I'm afraid I might be too nervous to nurse.

This is a fairly common worry, but isn't really a necessary one. All nursing mothers are not the same; they are not all easy-going. The hormones that are associated with breastfeeding may make you feel surprisingly relaxed.

Also, you can do certain things that will help you to relax before each feeding. If you're more comfortable by yourself, go into another room to nurse. Lie on a bed, use a rocking chair to nurse, watch TV, or listen to music. Look forward to nursings as a time to put your feet up and to relax. Have something to drink, such as juice, water, or an occasional glass of beer or wine. Take a few deep breaths as you put the baby to the breast.

8. Do I have to be on a special diet while I am nursing?

No. You need to eat a well-balanced diet, with slightly larger amounts of protein foods and calcium. Most women eat slightly larger portions of the foods than they would normally be eating. If you do not eat properly, your milk will not dry up but you will be making milk at the expense of your own needs. You will not feel as well as you will if your diet is balanced and contains enough calories.

It is not necessary to drink milk; cheese and other dairy products are also good sources of calcium. Large amounts of some foods may bother some nursing babies. If certain foods such as cabbage or beans or orange juice make you feel uncomfortable, they may make your baby uncomfortable too.

Most women eat their usual diet and are unaware of any effects on the baby from what they eat.

9. My mother (or mother-in-law) is coming to help out when the baby is born. She bottle fed her babies. Will this make any difference?

If you feel more comfortable nursing when you are alone, nurse in a separate room.

People whose experience is only with bottle feeding sometimes have difficulty understanding the baby's need to nurse every 2½ hours. They may remark that the baby is always nursing, and be surprised by the erratic and frequent feeding schedule.

If your mother (or mother-in-law) tried unsuccessfully to nurse, she probably is not a source of good breastfeeding information. It seems to be human nature for people to subconsciously try to discourage others from undertaking or accomplishing something in which they failed or which they found difficult. (9).

10. Will I be able to nurse just as well if I have a cesarean delivery?

Yes. The birth of the baby and the placenta are what trigger the hormonal changes necessary for the onset of lactation in the first week postpartum. This happens whether the baby is delivered vaginally or by a cesarean section.

During the first day or two after a cesarean delivery a nurse can help you to position the baby comfortably at the breast.

11. Is it necessary to do nipple preparation?

Not unless you have flat or inverted nipples, in which case you should do the Hoffman technique and wear a milk cup. It is wise to avoid soap or other drying agents on your nipples during pregnancy and after the baby is born.

12. Can all women succeed at breastfeeding?

It is estimated that between 96% and 99% of all women can breastfeed. The most important factor in successful breastfeeding is simply wanting to nurse. Finding help and support from those who are familiar with breast-feeding can also help. Reading about breastfeeding during pregnancy is another positive step.

13. What about breast care creams?

Creams are not routinely needed on the nipple while pregnant or while breastfeeding. Natural lubrication is supplied by the tiny Montgomery glands. These glands are on the pigmented (darker) skin around the nipple and give a rough or "pimply" look to the area around the nipple. They are most noticeable when a woman is cold.

If your skin is very dry during pregnancy or while you are breastfeeding, you may need additional lubrication. Eucerin cream is available without a prescription from a pharmacist; it does not contain a long list of ingredients, as do some brand-name breast creams, and it is also cheaper. Apply the cream in a thin coat around, but not on the end, of the nipple once or twice a day.

14. Is it worthwhile to breastfeed if I have to go back to work?

Yes. Even if you have to go back as early as six weeks, you can nurse while you are at home with your baby. A lot of women do this. You can plan to wean your baby to a bottle before you go back to work, or you can plan to continue nursing him in the morning and at night. It is up to you. You can make up your mind as you go along. Be sure your baby will accept a bottle if you must go back in the early weeks or months. The longer that you are able to take as maternity leave, the better it will be. If you are able to take six months, you can easily breastfeed without being concerned about bottles. By the end of that time, the baby will be able to use a cup. (see Chapter 11.)

15. How will I be able to sit and relax with my other children running around? How will my older children react to my nursing the baby?

If the parents accept breastfeeding as a natural and pleasant way to feed a baby, the other children will too. It may take some children a day or two to get used to the sight of their mother nursing—simply because of the more general acceptance of bottle feeding.

There are things you can do to help, such as involving an older child with the nursing. Spread out a blanket or old quilt so that the young child can be next to you while you nurse. Read a book to the older child while you nurse and have a snack of juice or cheese and crackers ready.

16. What about DDT, the PCBs, PBBs, etc.?

Concern about these chemicals often is related to mothers' milk in the newspapers and on television. The chemicals have been found in mothers' milk because they are found in our air, our water, in the food we eat. The real answer is for us to stop using such dangerous and persistent chemicals, not to stop breastfeeding.

In reports of chemicals in breast milk, one fact is repeated: the proven advantages of breastfeeding outweigh any theoretical dangers from chemicals that may be in the milk. There have been no demonstrated cases of harm to nursing babies. No responsible agency has recommended the widespread testing of human milk. The only women who are thought to have milk with potentially dangerous levels of contamination are women in special circumstances—those living on farms in Michigan where PBBs were inadvertently mixed with cattle feed, women who work in industries that have been exposed to high levels of chemical contamination, etc. (See Chapters 3 and 11.)

17. What about breastfeeding groups?

La Leche and other local groups have helped a lot of women learn about breastfeeding. Some women are very grateful to the groups. Other women find groups less appealing. The only way for you to know how you feel is to go to a meeting and see. Pregnancy is a good time to attend a meeting.

References

1.   Helsing, E: Lactation Education: The Learning of the "Obvious". CIBA Foundation Symposium no. 45:215, 1976.

2.   Dick-Read, G: *Childbirth Without Fear.* New York: Harper & Row, 1972.

3.   Hytten, FE and Baird, D: The development of the nipple in pregnancy, Lancet 1:1201, 1958.

4.   Hoffman, JB: Suggested treatment for inverted nipples, Am. J. Obstet. Gynecol. 66: 346, 1953.

5.   Otte, MJ: Correcting inverted nipples-an aid to breast feeding, Amer. J. Nurs. 75:454, 1975.

6.   Waller, H: The early failure of breastfeeding: a clinical study of its causes and their prevention, Arch. Dis. Child. 21(1), 1946.

7.   Brown, MS and Hurlock, JT: Preparation of the breast for breastfeeding, Nurs. Res. 24: 448, 1975.

8.   La Leche League International: The Womanly Art of Breastfeeding. Franklin Park, Illinois: LLL, 1963 and 1978 editions.

9.   Haire, D: The Nurse's Contribution to Successful Breast-feeding and the Medical Value of Breast-feeding. Chapter V of *Implementing Family Centered Maternity Care,* International Childbirth Education Association, 1974.

10. Eiger, MS and Olds, S: *The Complete Book of Breastfeeding.* New York: Workman Publishing & Co., Inc. 1972.

11. Jhirad, A and Vago, T: Induction of labor by breast stimulation, Obstet. Gynecol. 41:347, 1973.

12. La Leche League International: Leaven 8 (5), 1972.

Chapter 6

The Hospital Stay

GENERAL DISCUSSION

The events surrounding the birth of a child and the manner in which they are handled significantly affect early parent-infant interactions. The woman during labor and delivery is very sensitive to her surroundings. To a certain extent this sensitivity continues through the early postpartum days. Unspoken as well as spoken messages from anyone with whom the woman is in contact are taken personally and with extreme seriousness. A remark, even a casual comment, about the baby and nursing may be taken as a serious criticism; a simple word of praise may be reassuring out of proportion. The new mother's task during these days is to begin learning how to be a mother, how to breastfeed. She may not know the simplest skills, such as diapering, burping, and dressing a young infant. The maternity nurse who gives the new mother confidence in her own ability to do these things is best serving the mother's needs. Certainly there is no area where giving confidence to new mothers is more crucial than in breastfeeding. Helping the mother to relax and to enjoy nursing her baby should be a major goal of the nurse during the postpartum stay. After the first 24 hours following a normal delivery, most women require only minimal medical supervision. Unlike other hospital patients, they are not ill. So the remaining two or three days of the hospital stay are an ideal time to help them begin to learn mothering and breastfeeding skills.

It often is helpful to warn new mothers about the likelihood of intense feelings during the early days postpartum. In addition to being uncomfortable with constipation, hemorrhoids, and a healing episiotomy, many women experience extremes in mood, with periods of happiness alternating with inexplicable weepiness. It is helpful for the new mother to know that such feelings are common and transient.

The complete peace of a newborn baby comforted at the breast soon after birth is strong encouragement to a new mother (1). It is evidence of her ability to give total care to her newborn. Whenever possible, the first feeding experience of a new mother should be early and at the breast.

LABOR AND DELIVERY

Optimally, the mother is awake and alert through labor and delivery; father, or someone close to the mother, is present throughout to give her emotional support. Ideally, the parents are well-informed about the course of childbirth and are familiar with the hospital and its routines. When maternal anaesthesia is needed, regional or local anaesthesia is now recognized as preferable to general anaesthesia, sedative or centrally depressant agents. Minimum effective doses of analgesics should be used and only those agents with short half-life and the least effect on the alertness of the newborn child (2).

Proper   preparation during the last months of pregnancy can help to educate expectant parents about childbirth and about the risks and benefits of maternal analgesia. Ideally they can learn techniques to help make childbirth possible with as little medication as possible. Obviously they should be made to understand that analgesia is available and will be offered.

The infant born to a relaxed mother who has been awake and alert through labor and delivery is more likely at birth to be alert and responsive. After a normal delivery the child can immediately be offered to the parents for a period of privacy of at least 45-60 minutes. During this early contact many women will want to, and can be encouraged to, nurse their newborn (see below).

The existence of a "sensitive period" in the first hours after birth is indicated by recent observations of the effect of early parent-infant interactions on later behaviors (3). There is evidence that during this early period the infant is "bonding" to his mother (father). Klaus and Kennell hypothesize that through "reciprocal interactions," mother and infant reinforce within each other behaviors that guarantee feelings of love and satisfaction in the mother and security and comfort within the newborn. This promotes a continuing desire within the mother to hold, cuddle, love and nurse her infant. Similar emotional bonds occur between father and infant in the first hours and days.

The significance of bonding and the possibility of an early optimal sensitive period is demonstrated by studies comparing groups of new mothers given early intimate contact versus those with the traditional glance at the baby at birth and then brief contact six to eight hours later and then every four hours for feeds. Mothers given extended early contact within the first 12 hours tended to show more affectionate behavior to the infant in the hospital and on follow up evaluation (4). In several studies, more prolonged breastfeeding was noted in early contact groups (3). In addition, close early contact with the mother allows the immunologic protection of colostrum and the transfer of maternal bacterial flora (as against more pathogenic hospital flora).

The baby's alertness and ability to respond to his parents is affected by the management of labor and delivery. Babies born after general anaesthesia or after significant barbiturate sedation tend to be sleepy and less responsive. They may nurse ineffectively and infrequently during the first days of life (5). Although the effect is transient, it occurs at an important time. The baby who nurses poorly, who makes little eye to eye contact, who fails to respond to his mother's voice and movements, fails to reinforce her early mothering behaviors (3).

THE FIRST NURSING

In many cultures a newborn baby is put to his mother's breast or placed on the abdomen even before delivery of the placenta. It is a common response of a newly delivered mother to reach for her newborn. In the hospital setting, some women are not ready to hold and handle the baby immediately and are content to touch and then see their newborn placed in father's arms or held by a nurse for her to see. After the birth of the placenta and repair of any required episiotomy, the mother and baby can be brought to a labor, recovery, or postpartum room for a period of time alone together. Father or whoever has attended the mother through labor and delivery should be welcomed, however. In some hospitals, overhead heaters above the mother's bed are provided so that the baby can be undressed for this first meeting. This period of privacy can be interrupted for a first-time nursing mother, as she should be helped with the first nursing. Showing the mother how to position the baby and helping her to get started will be much appreciated. Often the newborn will not actually nurse, but will instead be satisfied to lick the mother's nipples. The mother can be reassured of the normalcy of this response. How the mother perceives this first nursing and subsequent early nursings can determine whether she will continue confidently with nursing rather than with hesitation and insecurity. Positive comments by the maternity nurse are extremely helpful in giving a new mother confidence.

Obviously this early nursing requires an undistressed baby and a mother who is awake and ready for her newborn (see Fig. 6-1).

The main lesson to be taught to the new mother in the first day is simply how to position her baby at the breast. She may be reassured that all moth-

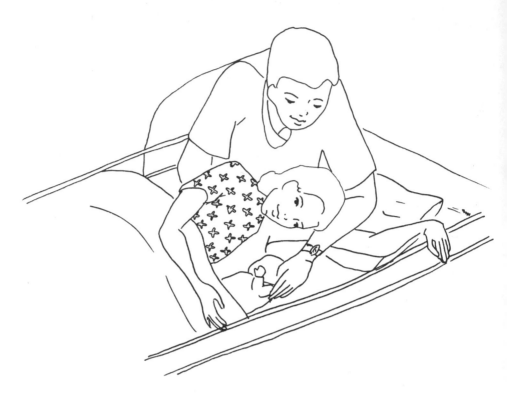

Figure 6-1. Mother, baby, and father at the first feeding.

ers find it awkward the first time. Regardless of what nursing position is used, all correct nursing positions have these points in common: [1] The mother is truly comfortable; her arms, shoulders and legs are supported and relaxed. She is in a position that one could comfortably maintain for a considerable time. The nervous new mother who tends to hunch her shoulders or who leans over the baby needs help in finding a comfortable position. In many cases one or two pillows may be helpful. [2] The baby's whole body is rotated toward the mother's body (see Fig. 6-2). Normally, the gaze of the mother and the gaze of the baby are directed toward one another: mother and baby are *en face*.

THE POSTPARTUM UNIT

The new mother usually is brought to a postpartum unit following a variable period of recovery. Rooming-in with the mother taking full care of her infant with the ready help of maternity staff soon after delivery is most desirable. A full examination of the normal newborn is customary within the

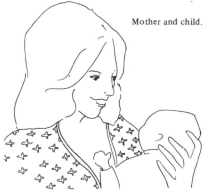

Mother and child.

a) The mother gets to know the baby prior to putting him to the breast.

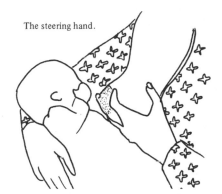

The steering hand.

b) The hand guides the mother's nipple well back into the baby's mouth *after* triggering the rooting reflex.

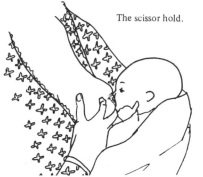

The scissor hold.

c) The scissor hold keeps the mother's breast away from the baby's nose so that he can breathe easily while nursing.

Figure 6-2.
Scenes at the First
Nursing.

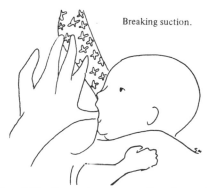

Breaking suction.

d) The little finger breaks suction to end the nursing.

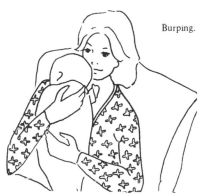

Burping.

e) The mother burps the baby before offering the second breast.

first 24 hours of birth and can, whenever possible, be done in mother's presence. The joy of telling a new mother that her newborn child is beautiful and perfect is one of the real pleasures of being a pediatrician or family doctor. New mothers need encouragement that all is well.

THE PHYSICIAN'S ORDERS IN THE NURSERY

Routine orders usually include provision for vitamin K, $AgNO_3$ eye drops, and feeding orders. The nursing mother should be encouraged to nurse on a demand schedule from the very start. Ordering a period of nothing by mouth after birth should not be necessary if the baby is born with little or no systemic maternal analgesia or systemic anaesthetic. The use of a first feed of water or glucose water also is unnecessary. Obviously the newborn who is distressed in any way may well need special observation and withholding of feeds may be appropriate. Obviously, if there is suspicion of tracheo-esophageal fistula (hydramnios, excessive mucous secretions), further tests are essential prior to beginning feeds. Tracheo-esophageal fistual is estimated to occur in 1 in 3,000 births (6).

Daily weights should be ordered and checked for excessive losses. If nursing is started early and continued frequently on a demand basis, approximately every 2-2½ hours, weight loss often is minimal. The usually accepted 10% weight loss over the first week represents a slow acquisition of adequate milk supply. Weight loss is less when frequent nursing is encouraged.

If a large weight loss does occur, there should be prompt investigation of nursing routines. An attempt to increase the number of nursings often is all that is required. Sometimes water supplements are needed—such as when weight loss is excessive and a trial of increased nursing is not yet successful, or when bili-lights are required.

Water or glucose water supplements, when occasionally needed, should be offered only after nursings and, less frequently, perhaps after every other nursing. Using a spoon or dropper instead of a bottle has been suggested to avoid confusion between suckling at the breast and sucking on a rubber nipple. It is inappropriate to order formula supplements. Since the PKU test is reliable only when feeding is established, the test should be repeated at the two week check up.*

If mother is unable to have rooming-in, breastfeeding should begin as soon as she feels ready and should continue, if she is able, on at least an every three hours schedule during the day. Optimally the baby can be

---

* One recent study has suggested that repeat PKU tests are not actually picking up missed cases (in the United States). It should be noted, however, that because of low levels of phenylalinine in breast milk, the totally breastfed infant may be more difficult to screen early on (7). Further study is needed to determine the best screening policy.

brought to mother when he first awakens and can, in this way, be kept on close to a demand schedule. Obviously, at times this may not be possible. A demand schedule avoids prolonged periods of the newborn crying in the nursery followed by the frustration of having a baby who is too tired to nurse. One or two night nursings should also be given.

Common breast problems such as soreness and engorgement are discussed in Chapter 8. Devices such as shields and bottles are discussed in Chapter 14.

THE EDUCATION OF NEW MOTHERS ON THE POSTPARTUM UNIT

In many cases most of the information that mothers ever receive about breastfeeding is given in the three or four days spent in a postpartum unit, and much of it is given by the nurses. Although consistency in information has often been cited as ideal for new mothers who are learning about breastfeeding, differences of opinion on breastfeeding techniques are still sometimes found on maternity wards, such as over the use of shields and bottles, the exact duration of feedings, the use of heat versus cold for engorgement. Ensuring that the information on a maternity floor is basic and consistent may be effected most easily through some form of in-service education.

In-Service Training of Health Professionals

If nearly all healthy babies are rooming-in, the central nursery is likely to be relatively empty for much of the day. The focus for the nursery nurses thus can change from primarily caring for infants to teaching new mothers. (It has been noted that such a change is not always welcome to some who have enjoyed tending and feeding babies.) Experienced and inexperienced nurses alike will function even more effectively as teachers of breastfeeding mothers if they themselves have received instructions in the specifics, as can be covered in an in-service on breastfeeding techniques.

The person who conducts an in-service on techniques should emphasize that, ideally, when there is time to give breastfeeding information to mothers, the information should be *basic, consistent,* and *preparatory for the first days at home.*

The Characteristics Of Helpful Breastfeeding Information

1. *Basic.* Above all, it should be pointed out at an in-service that breastfeeding is not instinctive but needs to be taught—ideally, throughout the 3-4 day hospital stay. The teaching should include, in addition to help in positioning the baby at the breast, information that promotes an understanding of lactation. Such basic information includes:

(a) Supply and demand: the more the baby nurses, the more milk there will be.

(b) Newborns nurse frequently, on the average of 10 times each 24 hours.

(c) Feedings are a good time to relax and to enjoy a new baby.

Clearly, the above are simple ideas, easy to explain, and vital to successful lactation. Peripheral information, such as nipple care routines and advice about fluid intake or bras, should never be given to the exclusion of basic information.

2. *Consistent.* Consistent policies on the use of devices such as milk cups and shields, on the use of bottles, and on managing common problems such as engorgement and soreness can be explained. Everyone who comes in contact with the nursing mother should give consistent advice.

3. *Preparatory for the First Days at Home.* Although some preparatory teaching is ideally handled as discharge planning, the experience in the hospital also is vitally important and should be aimed at preparing the new mother for nursing after discharge from the hospital. Nowhere is the old cliche that actions speak louder than words more relevant than in a maternity unit. The mother's patterns of breastfeeding at home are often based on both what she *sees* and on what is told to her in the hospital. Impressionable new mothers often mimic hospital routines, which almost seem to be imprinted during the hospital stay. An example of this is given by Brazelton who notes the tendency of new parents to swaddle the newborn and place him on the right side at home "just like they did in the hospital." (8)

Although no bottles or shields of any kind are usually needed and may even interfere with the newborn's ability to suckle effectively, new mothers may assume that bottles or shields are needed routinely at home if they see them ever-present in the maternity unit. Emphasizing ounces lost-and-gained or clock-watching also is counter productive. Helpful remarks and practices in the hospital are those which encourage the mother to nurse according to the baby's needs while she is in the hospital and later at home. This will help new mothers to understand that nursing is comfort as well as nourishment.

At some point during the second or third day of the

mother's hospital stay, the advantage of varying the nursing position can be explained to the mother in terms that she can readily understand. "Would you like to try nursing sitting up? (or lying down?—whatever she has not yet tried) That way the same points on your nipples will not be stressed and become sore." The mother who resists the idea of varying the nursing position, and whose nipples are not becoming sore, may continue with her preferred position. Also, during the last days of the mother's hospital stay, it may be appropriate to give her suggestions to help her condition her let-down reflex to nursing such as by taking a drink of water, sitting in one comfortable place, or taking a few deep breaths just before each feeding. The normalcy of uterine contractions during nursings, especially in multiparous women, can be mentioned.

Free Formula and Pamphlets

It has been common practice to give breastfeeding mothers a pamphlet prepared by a formula manufacturer and sometimes a free sample of formula. These pamphlets most often contain misleading information (i.e., feeding every 3-4 hours) and/or peripheral (relatively unimportant) information. It is likely that a new mother reading such a pamphlet will feel doubly inadequate. She has finished reading a pamphlet, supposedly on how to breastfeed, but what she still does not know is how to breastfeed. The centerfold, which may contain a pretty and relaxed mother giving a "supplemental bottle" to her young infant, appears to equate confidence with bottle feeding. Lack of confidence by new mothers in their milk supply correlates highly with lactation failure and early weaning.

If printed materials are wanted, the hospital can purchase more proper inexpensive ones (see Appendix A) or it can print its own.

WHAT EVERY NEW NURSING MOTHER WANTS TO KNOW

Following are some questions commonly asked by new nursing mothers, and some suggested answers. Detailed discussions of some of the points appear in later chapters.

1. How often shall I nurse my baby?

Nursing on demand is ideal and will help make nursing easier and more relaxed. Nursing is comfort as well as food. It is easier to nurse an unhappy baby than to try to put off the feeding by walking, rocking or using other "stalling tactics." Newborn babies normally nurse frequently, every one and a half to three hours.

2. How long should I nurse?

First nursings are probably best kept to 5 to 10 minutes per breast. There is a lot of disagreement on this point, but keeping first nursings brief may avoid some nipple soreness. (See Chapter 8) As long as your nipples are comfortable, you may gradually increase the length of feedings. If soreness begins to develop, it is best to limit nursings to 5 minutes/breast. Be sure to air-dry nipples after each feeding. Gradually lengthen feeding times, trying to nurse approximately the same time on each breast. Vary the nursing positions.

3. Should I be doing anything special to my nipples?

Yes, and no. Avoid soap and other drying agents. Nipples need not be washed before or after feedings; plain water during a daily bath is sufficient cleaning. Bra pads with plastic linings should be avoided, especially during the first weeks. Air drying after feeds is most important in keeping the nipple skin healthy. Breast creams are not needed unless the skin is excessively dry; they can be detrimental to macerated skin. If a cream is used, use it sparingly.

4. Should I wear a bra?

If you are more comfortable with one, yes. Some women prefer not to wear a bra. Wearing a bra that is too tight is definitely harmful. It is better to use a bra extender or remove the bra.

5. What can I do for engorgement?

Engorgement is best prevented by suckling frequently, day and night. When breasts are full, it is difficult for the baby to grasp the nipple. (See Chapter 8) Engorgement disappears gradually over the first week, and this does not mean your milk is disappearing.

6. Should I give the baby water or supplements?

Ordinarily the breastfed baby needs no other nutrition or fluid in addition to breast milk. If you want to get the baby used to bottles, you may offer one occasionally. (See Chapter 14)

Classes

One way to ensure that mothers do learn basic information about breastfeeding is to hold informal classes on the postpartum unit. These may be given by a maternity nurse or lactation counselor. (See also Chapter 1)

The information should be consistent and should help to prepare the mother for going home.

ADVICE ON DISCHARGE

Most often mothers are discharged during the first week postpartum, often simultaneously with the milk coming in and before lactation really is established. Ensuring professional contact with a new mother during the first days at home may be vital to successful nursing. General advice that should be given to a mother prior to discharge (or may be given in printed handouts) might include the following:

. . . . .Checklist of Advice Upon Discharge . . . .

1.   The first day home from the hospital is usually stressful. There is tension in parents' learning new roles; newborns are often fussy.

2.   A period of fussinesss, usually in late afternoon or evening, is frequent in young infants and is usually not caused by hunger, a wet diaper, or anything else that is fixable by parents. The nursing mother should try not to equate this with inadequate milk supply or something being wrong with her milk.

3.   The baby who is wetting 6 or more diapers per day with dilute urine and who is content after nursing, who is being nursed on demand is most likely to be receiving sufficient milk.

4.   Newborns are unspoilable. Nurse on baby's demand, but especially encourage frequent day-time nursings (every 2-2½ hours, sometimes more often). An average of 8-12 feeds per 24 hours is normal. Remember, nursing is comfort as well as nutrition.

5.   Nighttime feeds are important to the milk supply, but many babies confuse day and night. By encouraging frequent feeds during the day, a mother can slowly decrease feeds at night.

At the time of discharge, advice on baby care can be given by the physician who will be caring for the baby and/or by the maternity nurse who is responsible for the mother's hospital discharge. It is important to ensure that someone is responsible for giving (in addition to advice on diaper rash, vitamins, etc.) some simple advice about nursing during the first days and weeks at home.

Confidence in her own ability to feed her baby is probably the most valuable asset a new mother can take home from her hospital stay.

References

1.   Gunther, M: The new mother's view of herself, in CIBA Foundation Symposium no. 45: 145, 1976.

2.   American Academy of Pediatrics Committee on Drugs: Effect of medication during labor and delivery on infant outcome, Pediatrics 62: 402, 1978.

3.   Klaus, MH and Kennell, JH: *Maternal-Infant Bonding.* St. Louis: C.V. Mosby Company, 1976.

4.   Sosa, R, Kennell, JH, et al.: The effect of early mother-infant contact on breastfeeding, infection and growth, CIBA Foundation Symposium no. 45:179, 1976.

5.   Brazelton, TB: Psychophysiologic reactions in the neonate. II. Effect of maternal medications on the neonate and his behavior affected by obstetric sedation, Pediatrics 37:1012, 1966.

6.   Behrman, RD: *Neonatology.* St. Louis: C. V. Mosby Company, 1973.

7.   Binder, J: Phenylketonuria in a breastfed child. Pediatrics 63:334, 1979.

8.   Brazelton, TB: *Infants and Mothers.* N.Y.: Dell Publishing Co., 1969.

Chapter 7

Complications in the Immediate Postpartum Period

This chapter discusses some relatively common complications of the postpartum period that may require special measures in breastfeeding management.

CESAREAN BIRTH

Breastfeeding is as appropriate after cesarean delivery as after normal delivery. In fact, breastfeeding may ease some of the feelings of disappointment after cesarean delivery in women who had anticipated a conscious cooperative childbirth.

The main obstacles to breastfeeding are the mother's discomfort and difficulty in maneuvering; therefore suggestions should be specific to enable her to position the baby comfortably at the breast and avoid the incision. It is appropriate to offer reassurance to any mother who has doubts that she can breastfeed, and to tell her that she may feel closer to her baby. She may need to be told that milk production is triggered by hormone changes following delivery and will not be adversely affected by a cesarean delivery. New mothers may not know this fact.

If it is the policy to place cesarean babies under observation or to put them in a special nursery, this should be explained to the mother so she will not assume there is something wrong with her baby. However, the practice is increasing (appropriately) of not immediately separating an undistressed newborn from his parents at birth, especially if mother was awake during the delivery. If the baby is sleepy because the mother was given general anaesthesia, the mother should be reassured that this is to be expected.

The mother should be given confidence that she will feel more comfortable and competent and find nursing more enjoyable as the days pass. A sleepy baby will nurse better in time as the effects of anaesthesia wear off, but this may take several days. How soon after delivery the baby is first brought to suckle depends on hospital policy and the condition of the mother. In many cases the mother can be allowed to nurse and to be with her baby immediately after delivery and completion of surgery, usually in a recovery room.

Many cesarean mothers first nurse lying on their sides, with pillows for support. The nurse places the baby, lying on his side, with his mouth next to the mother's nipple. When the nipple touches the baby's cheek he will root and take the nipple into his mouth. When it is time for the second breast, the mother can be helped by the nurse to turn on to her other side. The nurse can then position the baby at the second breast. The side rail on the bed can help the mother to support herself and to turn. As with non-cesarean mothers, nursing should be encouraged as early as possible.

For later feedings some cesarean mothers find that they are more comfortable sitting up to nurse. A pillow on the lap to protect the incision and raise the baby up to the level of the breast is important. Some women prefer to alternate this position with the football hold, which directs the baby's legs away from the incision. If rooming-in is not possible, the physician's orders should encourage feeds every three hours as soon as mother is able.

The cesarean mother needs to be encouraged to rest at home when she is leaving the hospital, and breastfeeding is clearly compatible with resting.

Some childbirth groups in the United States have a special support group for cesarean mothers. There is an organization called C/SEC, Inc. which provides information on cesarean births and can furnish a list of local organizations. (See Appendix A)

JAUNDICE IN THE BREASTFED INFANT

Breast milk jaundice is a distinct clinical entity characterized by prolonged unconjugated hyperbilirubinemia, associated with breast milk feedings in the young infant (1,2). This is estimated by one source to occur with a frequency of about one in 200 breastfed babies and to recur in three-fourths of an affected woman's future breastfed infants (1). The importance of recognizing this syndrome lies in differentiating it from other causes of hyperbilirubinemia.

Infants with breast-milk jaundice are asymptomatic in the first days of life. Jaundice occurs coincident with the onset of milk "coming-in", usually on the 4th or 5th day. Peak levels of unconjugated bilirubin between 15 and 25 mg% occur during the second or third weeks of life. Even if nursing is continued, these levels gradually decrease to normal over a period of days to weeks. Levels of bilirubin above 15 mg% should be treated with withdrawal of breast milk. Also this may help confirm the diagnosis: the diagnosis of breast milk jaundice is made by stopping the breastfeeding for a short period (24-48 hours) to document a coincident fall in bilirubin level. When nursing is resumed, there is usually a rise in bilirubin level again, but often to a much lower level. Nursing can then be continued and mother reassured that the jaundice is benign in nature and is not an indication for cessation of nursing. Bilirubin levels can continue to be followed as long as necessary. The mother should be informed of the expected length of the jaundice period. There is no need to prescribe formula supplements or to limit nursing.

The etiology of breast-milk jaundice may involve multiple factors (2,3,4, 5). It was originally believed to be related to the presence of pregnane-3α20 βdiol (gestational progesterone) in the breast milk of affected women. This substance in vitro is an inhibitor of liver glucuronyl transferase (an enzyme necessary for bilirubin metabolism) and is found in the milk and urine of mothers with infants with the syndrome but does not always correlate with jaundice clinically. Other factors such as increased levels of certain free fatty acids in the affected breast milk (e.g., linoleic acid), as well as factors peculiar to each child (e.g., relative maturity of liver enzyme system) are other possible causes.

Serum bilirubins of greater than 2.0 mg% occur in most term newborn infants, with peak values of about 6-8 mg% occurring between the third to sixth day of life. These elevated levels of bilirubin (mostly unconjugated bilirubin) are believed to be due to the combination of a relatively immature liver and an increased bilirubin load present from birth. The increased bilirubin load is caused by the shorter life span of red blood cells in early infancy and to the greater absorption of bilirubin from the newborn's gut. The newborn's liver is, in the first days of life, less efficient at bilirubin uptake and additionally there is decreased activity of the liver enzyme glucuronyl transferase, which is necessary for metabolism of bilirubin.

This "physiological" jaundice is a transient jaundice which usually begins to disappear in the term infant by the end of the first week. Normal bilirubin values occur by the end of the second week.

If there is extensive bruising or hematoma at birth, bilirubin levels are likely to be higher. In such infants, there is frequently need for treatment with phototherapy. Poor feeding with decreased fluid intake may occur with elevated bilirubin levels. When this occurs, water supplements after nursing are appropriate. This is no reason to stop nursing.

Physiological jaundice occurs in both breast- and bottle-fed infants.There is a tendency to over-diagnose breast milk jaundice in nursing babies with physiological jaundice. A 3 or 4 day old term baby with a rising unconjugated bilirubin is unlikely to have breast milk jaundice. The diagnosis here is mostly likely physiological jaundice and appropriate studies and management should be ordered. It is inappropriate to discontinue breastfeeding. If phototherapy is required, nursing can be continued, but placed on a schedule of only every three hours. If there is excessive water loss while under the bililights, water can be offered between nursings.

The ill or premature infant is likely to be in a special nursery and will require treatment of hyperbilirubinemia at lower levels than the term infant. Restrictions on nursing will depend on the child's other problems.

Diagnoses to be Considered in a
. . . . Jaundiced Newborn . . . .

1.   Physiologic jaundice

2.   Breast milk jaundice

3.   Hemolysis
       a. Blood group incompatabilities (e.g. Rh, ABO)
       b. Hemolytic anemias (e.g. hereditary spherocytosis, G6PD)
       c. Hematoma

4.   Genetic disorders of bilirubin metabolism
       a. Glucuronyl transferase deficiency
          type I: Criger-Najjar Syndrome (severe jaundice occuring in first days which persists; autosomal recessive inheritance)

          type II: An autosomal dominant disorder characterized by mild jaundice which may appear only in adolescence but which should be considered if breast milk jaundice is excluded in cases of prolonged unconjugated jaundice

       b. Transient familial neonatal hyperbilrubemia (6): rare syndrome of severe jaundice in first days of life, often requiring exchange transfusions and caused by an inhibitory substance in maternal and infant plasma which disappears spontaneously

5.   Infection
       a. Sepsis
       b. Urinary tract infection
       c. Toxoplasmosis, cytomegalic inclusion disease, congeital rubella, hepatitis

6. Liver disease
    a. Hepatitis
    b. Biliary atresia
    c. Galactosemia
    d. Reaction to drugs (e.g. vitamin K_3)

7. Other diagnoses
    a. Hypothyroidism
    b. Down's Syndrome
    c. Pyloric stenosis, intestinal obstruction

THE NEWBORN WHO WILL NOT NURSE

The problem of the newborn who when put to the breast either will not nurse or nurses very poorly is a frustrating one to the new mother. What is wrong and what can be done?

Problems Originating with the Infant

Does the problem lie with the infant? Is he sleepy from labor and delivery medications, is he premature or small for date, does he have Down's Syndrome or another physical problem? The infant's own best times of peak alertness should be used for nursings. He can be "jack-knifed" before feedings, if he appears sleepy. (Fig. 7-1)

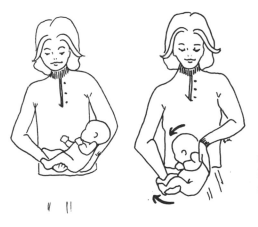

Figure 7-1. Jack-knifing.

Instructions: Support the infant's legs with one hand and his head and upper back with the other. Hold the baby supported lying on his back. Bring your two hands up and together, to bring the baby to a propped sitting position. Repeat gently 15 to 30 times just before a feeding to stimulate the infant.

According to Applebaum:

This simple Valsalva maneuver increases cardiac output and oxygen transport to the infant's brain, thereby increasing arousability, promoting strong sucking, and renewing the infant's interest at the breast. The mother may also express into the mouth of a too sleepy infant by compressing the areola between the fingers of her steering hand, a technique that is simlar to hand-expressing milk. In this way, a sleepy, poorly sucking infant may receive an extra ounce or two of milk with little active effort. The holding arm should push the head toward the chest simultaneously with each pumping compression so as to prevent the infant from pulling off the areola. (7)

If the baby seems to be sucking his own tongue, instead of suckling at the breast, he may need to be "reprogrammed" to suck properly by sucking on a Nuk Exercisor (pacifier) between feedings (8). Also, before each feeding the mother should use the rooting reflex in order to encourage the infant to open his mouth. The mother should watch his tongue to see that it is not up against the roof of the mouth before putting her nipple into the baby's mouth. Bottles should be avoided.

If the infant is crying, he should be calmed before being offered the breast.

The baby who is sleepy from maternal medications can be expected to spontaneously improve as the medications are metabolized in the first days postpartum.

Problems Originating with the Mother

The problem may be originating with the mother. Is she using incorrect feeding techniques, does she have poorly protractile nipples or engorgement?

The mother should be instructed in correct nursing techniques. She should be observed tactfully. She may need to learn how to depress her full breast with one hand so the infant's nose is not blocked. It may help to have her use one or two pillows to raise the infant to the level of her breasts. The baby should be placed lying on his side, facing the mother's rib cage and breast. The mother can hold the baby in the proper position by supporting his head in the crook of her arm. In cases of non-protractile nipples, corrective measures should be taken.(See Chapter 8)

Problems Caused by External Factors

The infant's refusal to nurse or his nursing poorly may be caused by external circumstances. Is the baby being brought to the mother on a fixed schedule; is the baby tired from crying; is the baby alternately being offered the breast and bottles of formula or water?

The routine is to eliminate any of the factors that may interfere with successful breastfeeding.

The recommendations for helping a woman to nurse an uncooperative baby are very similar to the recommendations for any mother and baby. The following measures were recommended in a commentary of the American Academy of Pediatrics (9):

1.   Decrease the amount of sedation and/or anaesthesia given to the mother during labor and delivery.
2.   Avoid separation of the mother from her infant during the first 24 hours.
3.   Breastfed infants should be fed "on demand," rather than on a rigid 3-4 hour schedule. Discourage routine supplementary formula feedings.
4.   Provide the mother easy access to her infant; rooming-in is important to successful lactation.

THE PRE-TERM INFANT

Pre-term infants, those born prior to 38 weeks gestation, are increasingly being breastfed. The following table correlates mean gestation age with mean weight of the newborn.

. . . . Mean Intrauterine Weight*. . . . .

Gestational Age (weeks)	26	28	30	32	34	36	38
Weight (grams)	900	1100	1300	1600	2000	2500	3000

*Lubchenco et al, Ped. 37:403, 1966

Controversy exists about what the optimal nutrition is for the premature infant of less than 32-33 weeks gestation (10). Those that favor breast milk cite breast milk's specificity for the human infant, its easy digestability, and its lack of allergenicity. Although early studies of growth in premature infants seemed to show slower growth of pre-term infants on breast milk compared to those fed formula (11,12), the seeming greater growth in the moderately premature infant (34-38 weeks) on formula possibly is related to increased water retention in infants due to the increased electrolyte content of the formulas used and may not represent true body growth (12, 13). Most agree that the mildly to moderately premature infant grows as well on breast milk as on formula (12,14). However, the question of optimal nutrition for the extremely premature infant, the infant less than 32 to 33 weeks gestation, is more complicated because there is no known optimal growth rate for these infants. Many neonatologists have striven to attain the same growth rate expected were the baby still in utero. Using calculations of absolute body content of fetuses at various ages in gestation through term, it has been possible to estimate how much protein, sodium, calcium, potassium, etc., a baby acquires while in utero. Using these calculations it is possible to show that breast milk has insufficient quantities of protein, sodium, and calcium to maintain in utero growth rates in the extra utero very premature infant (15); all other nutrients and electrolytes are apparently in adequate supply. These studies depend on the previously mentioned unproven assumption that the in utero growth rate is the optimal growth rate for the immaturely born infant. These growth rates would require high protein concentrations in the preparation that is fed.

There is some evidence that such high protein feeds may be accompanied by certain metabolic derangements. In a study by Raiha et al. (16), growth of infants from 28 to 36 weeks gestation was studied. All received the same absolute caloric intake. Five groups of infants were studied. Four groups were fed formula as follows: [1] a 1.5 g% protein formula with whey: casein ration of 60:40; [2] a 3.0 g% protein with whey:casein of 60:40; [3] a 1.5 g% protein with whey:casein of 18:82; and [4] a 3.0 g% protein with whey:casein of 18:82. The fifth group received pooled breast milk.

All five groups had similar growth rates within similar gestational age groups. However, significant abnormalities in blood urea nitrogen, urine osmolarity, and blood ammonia occurred in those fed higher protein formula. Metabolic acidosis was present in many of the formula-fed infants and also correlated with the higher protein formula; metabolic acidosis correlated also with the whey to casein ration of 18:82. Elevated amino acids were found in the serum of both high-protein formula fed groups. The group fed the low protein formula with the whey:casein of 60:40 was least dissimilar metabolically to the breast milk group (17,18). The limited ability of the preterm infant to convert methionine to cystine (making cystine an essential amino acid in the preterm baby) also was documented (19). This study questions findings of other studies which record faster growth with formulas of high protein (14) and also raises the question of safety of using high protein concentrations in infant feeds.

Recently the nitrogen content of milk of prematurely delivered women has been measured and is reportedly higher than that of the woman delivering at term. Both groups show a similar rate of decrease in concentration of protein with time (20). The clinical relevance of this finding is unclear at present, and further study is needed. The finding is, however, interesting and may be of clinical significance.

In addition to nutritional considerations for the premature infant, the question of immunological protection also may be a consideration. Clearly a major threat to survival in the preterm infant is infection. Protective factors in colostrum and breast milk would seem even more vital to the immature infant, but clinical human studies are not yet available. One study in rats demonstrated protection from necrotizing enterocolitis when either formula or maternal milk was fed, if live milk cells were included (21). This raises the question of persistence of cells and immunoglobulins in processed human milk. Heating causes loss of both cells and antibody activity; freezing destroys cells but spares immunoglobulins. Ideally, the premature infant who is to receive breast milk should receive his own mother's fresh breast milk. The possibility of a graft vs. host reaction to donor milk in the immunologically immature infant has been raised but has so far not been a clinical problem.

Perhaps some additional nutrients added to fresh human milk will be the answer to the question of optimal nutrition for the very premature infant. For now, the mother who wishes to express her milk for a small premature infant can be encouraged and helped to do so.

Healthy infants born at 36-38 weeks gestation usually will be able to suckle. Healthy infants born at 34-36 weeks gestation may or may not be able to suckle. It should be assumed that the mother of a premature infant who wants to breastfeed will require special help and encouragement. Once nursing is established, good weight gains can be expected. Successful breast-feeding mothers of premature infants find their nursing experience gratifying and worth the extra effort.

Nursing techniques effective for term infants are often ineffective with premature infants, and special instructions may be needed.

The premature baby who seems large and strong enough to be put to the breast still may not nurse well. The major problem is that premature babies fall asleep at the breast and may be too weak to nurse vigorously. The mother needs reassurance that, with patience and persistence, she will be able to nurse.

. . . . . Suggestions For Breastfeeding Premature Infants . . . . .

1. The mother who will be putting her small infant to the breast for the first time should be given instructions in proper positioning. The premature is likely to have more difficulty than a term baby in suckling at the breast and may be unable to keep hold of the mother's nipple; his head needs to be supported in the nursing position. Unlike a term baby who can turn his head to root, the premature should be held in such a way that his body is directed toward the mother's breast. One or two pillows can be placed on the mother's

lap; the baby can be placed lying on his side, facing the mother's rib cage and breast. The mother's arm can lay on the pillow, with her hand cupping the baby's buttocks. The crook of the mother's arm supports the baby's head and keeps it from flopping backward. The mother can use her free hand to guide the nipple to the baby's mouth and hold her breast so that his nose is not blocked (see the scissor hold Fig. 6-2).

2.   As with the term baby, the healthy premature ideally is, whenever possible, put to the breast directly, avoiding sucking confusion with bottle feeds. The first nursing can be initiated as soon as the physician has examined the infant and found him in sufficiently good condition.

3.   The mother should nurse very frequently, sometimes hourly. The feedings probably will be short, 2-3 minutes, as the baby tires easily and tends to fall asleep. Each mother will need to work out her own schedule with her baby. Some babies will awaken to nurse every two hours. The times of peak alertness by the infant should be taken advantage of for nursing; diaper changing and such can be done after the feeding. A baby who can nurse only very briefly on one breast should be awakened to nurse approximately once every hour. Rooming-in is appropriate for the healthy infant. The mother can be reassured that this schedule, which is difficult on her, will not last for very long. As the baby gains in strength, weight and maturity, he will be able to nurse on a schedule more like a full-term baby.

4.   The mother can try massage and hand-expression to get the milk flowing before putting the baby to breast.

5.   If the rooting reflex is weak, or appears to be absent, the mother will need to pull down on the baby's chin to get him to open his mouth, then put her nipple well back in the baby's mouth.

6.   Stroking the baby under the chin may encourage him to keep suckling.

7.   If the baby is sleepy, the mother should use different rousing techniques, such as jack-knifing (earlier in chapter) just before putting the baby to the breast.

8. Feeding the baby with parenteral fluids and/or tube feedings is often necessary initially for the immature or sick premature infant. With time these infants, if they survive, eventually graduate to bottle feeds. If the mother has been pumping her breasts to provide breast milk, she may eventually be allowed to put the baby to the breast. Many mothers have been unable to make this transition from expressing milk to nursing. The baby often does not nurse, having become accustomed to the bottle. There are suggestions to help these mothers and many will be successful if they are patient and persistent.

Measures to Encourage the
. . . . . . .Previously Bottle Fed Infant to Suckle . . . .

(a) The mother can encourage the baby to nurse while he is sleepy, just awakening, or can nurse him when he is not ravenously hungry. She should use her fingers to form her nipple and slip it into his mouth. If he will accept the mother's nipple at all, she can be encouraged to keep trying.

(b) Offering the breast as a pacifier, when the baby is not particularly hungry, may help the infant to accept the mother's nipple.

(c) Some mothers have found that expressing milk into the baby's mouth helped him to accept the breast.

(d) As a last resort the mother can put a small amount of sugar water* on the nipple or try using the all-rubber breast shield; the infant who is accustomed to the rubber of the bottle nipple may nurse through the shield. Because of the danger of having the baby then refuse to nurse without the shield, the mother should remove it after a few minutes. If this causes the baby to refuse to nurse, she can nurse with the shield, but cut it away gradually with a small pair of scissors, beginning from the center and cutting increasing amounts away before each feeding.

NURSING OF TWINS

The birth of twins is not a contraindication to breastfeeding for the mother who is interested. Mothers of twins are as likely to choose breastfeeding as are mothers of single-born babies (22). The woman who knows that she is

---

* Honey no longer can be advised because of an apparent association between it and botulism in the infant.

expecting twins, or who has recently given birth to twins, may require reassurance that she will be able to produce "enough milk," the ever-present question. Nearly all of the other vital points of information are the same as for a woman nursing one baby, that is, information on conditioning the let-down reflex, and the fact that milk production depends upon the amount of stimulation, "supply and demand." The key to nursing twins successfully lies in understanding breastfeeding concepts. Women who may have failed to nurse one baby often go on later to nurse twins after being given appropriate information and support (23). A mother who is beginning to nurse twins may be reassured by talking with another mother who has nursed twins (one may be found by contacting a breastfeeding-support group) or by reading about how to nurse twins (24).

If one or both twins must remain in the hospital after the mother is discharged, breastfeeding becomes more difficult, but still is possible. A mother may need to express her breast milk to maintain the supply. Expressed milk may be fed to hospitalized babies by tube or bottle. In some cases, the mother may be nursing one twin and expressing for the other.

After breastfeeding is established the mother's milk supply normally will be stimulated to keep pace with the babies' continuing demands. Growth spurts can be expected to occur with twins at approximately the same times as with single babies (10 days, 1 month, 3 months). The two babies may go through growth spurts, or periods of increased appetite, either at the same approximate time as each other or a week or more apart. More frequently, twins appear to go through the growth spurts one right after the other, so the combined growth spurt lasts for several days or a week. One week of very frequent nursings builds up the milk supply enough for two babies.

The question of nursing the two babies together or separately is one each mother has to decide for herself. Some mothers never feel comfortable nursing the two together and thus nurse each separately. Other mothers also find twin positioning somewhat awkward but feel they would never have any time left in the day unless they master a twin position.

Both babies can be held in the football hold with the support of pillows. One woman recommended sitting on a couch with many pillows so that both the mother's hands were free. This solves the problem that many mothers of twins mention: how do I get a baby repositioned if he wriggles out of place? (See Fig. 7-2 [a].)

Both babies can be nursed in the regular sitting-up position with one baby's legs across the other baby. In this case the mother can keep her hands on the babies' bottoms; when one wiggles, she can pull him back by grabbing the diaper. Again the mother needs pillows to support the babies (see Fig. 7-2 [b]).

One baby can be held in the football position with his body supported

Figure 7-2. Positions for nursing twins.

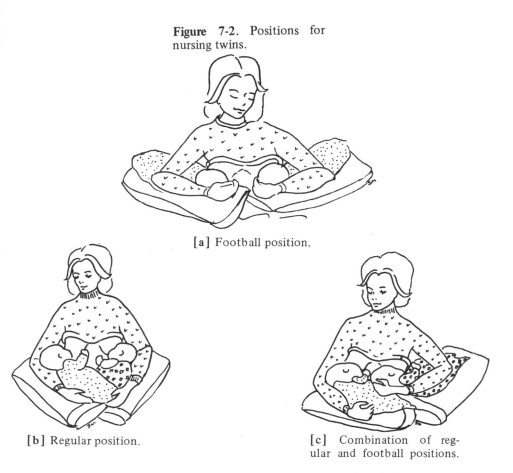

[a] Football position.

[b] Regular position.

[c] Combination of regular and football positions.

by a pillow and the other baby can be held in the regular sitting up position (see Fig. 7-2 [c]).

Some mothers nurse simultaneously for some feedings, when both babies have awakened at the same time, but separately for other feedings. If the mother wants to try nursing lying down, she can lie on her left side and nurse one baby on the left breast in the traditional lying-down position. The other baby can nurse on the right breast by lying across the mother's chest.

Should each twin have his own breast? In most cases where nursing continues for months, each twin does eventually have his own breast and the supply on each side adjusts to the amount of stimulation it is given. In the beginning, mothers are usually advised to swap the babies back and forth. In many cases one of the twins is a stronger sucker and can stimulate a better milk supply on both sides. If one of the twins was much smaller than the other, his nursing may be noticeably weaker.

The best general advice on the question of which side for which baby is this: nurse the hungriest baby on the fullest breast.

Scheduling: Many mothers find that they can cope best by following a modified demand schedule. The first twin awakens and needs to nurse. The mother can either awaken the second twin to nurse simultaneously, if she prefers to nurse the two together in order to save time; or, she can nurse the first twin and then, immediately after, awaken the second twin to nurse. Or both babies may be nursed on a demand schedule whenever they awaken (25).

The mother of twins may feel she needs to get away occasionally and therefore to use occasional bottles. Mothers of twins are sometimes surprised when asked if the use of bottles affects their supply; they feel their supply is super-abundant and occasional bottles do not create a problem.

The need for an excellent diet and for rest are obvious but not always easy for mothers of twins to manage. The mother is likely to be very thirsty and hungry.

There are two observations with twin nursing that may need additional study for clarification—problems in bonding, and an apparently higher incidence of mastitis.

Bonding with one of the two babies frequently appears to be more difficult, especially if one twin has had to remain in the hospital longer than the other or if one twin has more medical problems. The mother finds it natural to bond with one baby but not so with two at once. Klaus and Kennell describe clinical observations with twins and suggest that the phenomenon of mother-to-infant attachment is developed and structured so that a close attachment can optimally be formed to only one person at a time. Further, they report clinical observations of a much higher incidence of mothering disorders (battering, failure to thrive) with the second twin, who may have remained in the hospital nursery after the first twin was discharged. The clinical implication is that when possible the twins be kept together and discharged at the same time so that simultaneous attachments may be more likely (26).

The theory of bonding may explain observations about some new mothers of twins. Sometimes a mother may make what appear to be "silly excuses" for not visiting the second twin in the hospital, for not talking about the second twin, or not breastfeeding the second twin, while she is doing all those things for the first twin. Mothers have been observed to nurse one twin but refuse to try nursing the second twin.

With many mothers of twins, however, differences in bonding do not appear to be significant.

Another potential problem for the mother who is breastfeeding twins or triplets is an apparently higher incidence of mastitis. It is not clear exactly why the larger milk supply predisposes mothers to get infections, but this has been observed in many mothers of twins. The woman can be encouraged not to go for long periods without emptying the breasts and not to neglect her rest and diet.

Solids may not need to be introduced earlier than with single babies. When solids are introduced, most mothers use just one spoon and one dish of food and feed the babies at the same time. The mother spoons the food into twin A, while twin B swallows, and then the mother feeds B as A swallows. Then the feeding can be finished in as little time as for spoon-feeding one baby. Many mothers of twins rely heavily on finger foods.

Most mothers of twins find that unobtrusive double nursing is impossible in public and often nurse one baby at a time if someone else can be found to hold the other baby.

In cases of mother-led weaning, the mother weans both twins to bottles or cups at the same time. In cases of baby-led weaning, the twins often wean at different times, even several months apart.

Triplets

Feeding triplets is not easy, regardless of whether the mother breastfeeds or bottle-feeds. In both cases, the mother spends much of every day in feeding. In most cases the triplets are small prematures who must remain in the hospital for some time. It is not known if every mother can supply enough milk to completely nourish three babies. Many breastfeeding mothers of triplets prepare one batch of formula a day and take turns giving one of the three babies a bottle when all cannot be satisfied at the breast. Mothers often swap babies between the two breasts. Like mothers of twins, they either nurse two of them simultaneously, or nurse all separately.

CONGENITAL DEFECTS

In the case of congenital defects that do not directly affect breastfeeding, breastfeeding is clearly recommended for those women who want to do so. Because the mother is likely to be grieving for the perfect baby whom she had anticipated in her mind during pregnancy and whom she has lost, she may need time to go through a process of grieving. The mother who is coping with feelings of guilt, mourning, and grief, may find bonding more difficult (26). She may have difficulty in conditioning the let-down reflex. Time spent talking with the physician and nurses is valuable in answering questions and in allowing the parents an opportunity to feel supported and to accept the situation. Breastfeeding can be encouraged.

The situation is different for the woman who had decided on breast-feeding but who gives birth to an infant with anomalies that may be incompatible with continued life. Traditionally, the mother was told that breastfeeding was not advisable and was given medication to suppress lactation. Certainly, it is not appropriate for an outsider to suggest to the mother that she should breastfeed or provide expressed breast milk. Yet women have sometimes decided that they wanted to provide their own milk, despite the poor prognosis. Women have expressed breast milk for weeks for infants with serious heart defects, for example. As in the case of the premature infant, the prognosis sometimes is poor but not without hope. Showing optimism is indicated if there is any hope of survival, lest the parent begin to mourn prematurely. "There is no evidence that if a favorable prediction proves to be incorrect and the baby dies, the parents will be harmed by the early optimism. There is almost always time to prepare them before the baby actually dies. If he lives and the physician has been pessimistic, it is sometimes difficult for the parents to become closely attached after they have figuratively 'dug a few shovelfuls of earth.' " (26)

But if the infant dies? Whether the giving of her own milk makes the grief at the time of death more bearable or more unbearable is impossible to know. The reactions of those women who have expressed milk for an infant who subsequently died indicate that it may be inappropriate to try to shield women from lactation. The woman may find satisfaction in the fact that she was able to provide something unique for her baby and may feel that the experience was valuable to her psychologically.

A mother who gave birth to premature twins both of whom died, felt that giving her milk was important to her: "Even though I knew both my sons had a slim chance of surviving, I felt that providing my milk played an important part in maternal-infant bonding. Because our first son died shortly after birth, and I had little opportunity to touch or see him, it had been more difficult for me to work through grieving for him. Because our second son lived for 16 days and he did take my milk, my immediate grief was more intense when he died, but has been easier to work through. By choosing to express milk, I gained a sense of personal accomplishment." (27)

The grieving process may also be made easier when the parents have first accepted the reality of the baby's existence if they have held and touched him. If these concepts of bonding and grieving are followed, in helping the parents of an infant who may die, the mother who wants to give her own milk should not be discouraged.

DOWN'S SYNDROME

Breastfeeding for a woman who wants to nurse is not only advisable, but may be specifically beneficial, for a baby with Down's Syndrome.

. . Specific Advantages To Breastfeeding the Down's Infant . .

1.   Breast milk is optimal nutrition for a Down's Syndrome baby, just as it is for the normal baby.

2.   Down's babies have a greater than average number of illnessess and thus the immunologic advantages of breastfeeding may be beneficial.

3.   One of the most widespread problems among children and adults with Down's Syndrome is the tendency toward obesity; breastfeeding may help to prevent this (however, there are no data available).

4.   Breastfeeding brings special feelings of closeness to the mother and baby. Breastfeeding can help the mother to feel tenderness and to feel close to the baby as quickly as posible. Breastfeeding, especially at times of let-down, can help the mother to find some degree of peace and emotional acceptance when she also may be facing possible feelings of guilt. This has been the report from many women. (28)

5.   Down's Syndrome babies tend to be too placid, and they may benefit from the touching and holding and skin contact connected with breastfeeding.

However, there are obstacles to the successful breastfeeding of Down's Syndrome babies. The feelings of depression, guilt, grief or disbelief can make a new mother question whether she should keep the baby, let alone nurse him. Down's Syndrome babies can learn to nurse, but in the beginning, it takes a great deal of time and patience to get the baby to nurse well at the breast. Some Down's babies have more difficulty than others in nursing. In general, the Down's baby is an extremely placid baby who has poor muscle tone. His mouth does not seem to be up to the task of suckling; his tongue hangs limply in the way. The baby should be held in a nursing position such that he is propped sitting up, if he has been falling asleep when he is lying down. The biggest initial problem in nursing is rousing the baby enough to nurse.

Arousal Techniques
The following techniques can be tried before or during an attempt to nurse the Down's Syndrome infant (or any sleepy infant). Mothers of infants with neurological problems comment that they often needed to alternate different rousing techniques for maximum effectiveness.

. . . . Arousal Techniques . . . .

1.   *Jack-knifing* (see the discussion earlier in this chapter)

2.   *Waking* the infant to nurse, persistently.

3.   *Increased handling,* body contact and skin contact, not leaving the baby alone in the crib.

4.   *Alternating rousing techniques,* such as putting a little cool water on the baby, undressing the baby, loosening the blankets around him, changing his diaper, giving him a bath.

5.   *Stroking* under the chin. If the infant falls asleep fairly soon after being put to the breast, the mother can stroke him under the chin as he nurses. The stroking motion is from the area over the back of the throat, forward to the chin, and is gentle but firm.

The mother may need to hand-express milk into the baby's mouth, or in more difficult cases, hand-express or pump the milk and give it to him via a cup or eye dropper, squirted into the corner of his mouth. As a last resort her milk can be given in a bottle. This mother has a problem: she doesn't want the baby to give up trying to nurse because the bottle is easier. Yet the baby must have nourishment. Many Down's Syndrome babies tend to be very slow gainers in the early weeks, especially if the baby is not able to nurse vigorously.

Even after jack-knifing, the mother may not be able to elicit a rooting reflex. If stroking the baby's cheek does not lead him to root or open his mouth, the mother will need to put her nipple into his mouth. She should compress her areola between two fingers (scissor hold) and gently pull down on the baby's chin to open his mouth. She cannot count on the baby to latch on. She may need to place her nipple well back in his mouth. She can use rousing techniques as needed. If the infant tends to sleep for long intervals, the mother must be persistent and patient in encouraging him to nurse.Regardless of the feeding method, many Down's Syndrome babies gain weight slowly.

Parents of Down's Syndrome infants may be informed of groups that are concerned with Down's Syndrome (see Appendix C).

CLEFT LIP OR PALATE

Traditionally it has been assumed that a baby born with either a cleft lip or palate or both cannot breastfeed because such a baby finds it difficult or impossible to form a seal around the mother's nipple and to maintain the suction needed to keep the nipple back in the baby's mouth. However, sometimes breastfeeding is feasible. But because it is still widely believed that it is impossible, very few mothers of babies with clefts initiate breastfeeding and thus the pool of experience is limited.

Although breastfeeding a baby with one or more clefts is often difficult, bottle feeding such a baby is also difficult and also requires extra time and patience. Slow weight gain and/or failure to thrive are not uncommon in these infants.

Cleft Lip

A baby who is born with one or more clefts in the lip, but with an intact palate often can nurse. If a mother has decided during pregnancy that she wants to nurse her baby, she can be told that this is possible. The mother will need help in adjusting to her baby's problem, but can be encouraged to try to breastfeed.

The specifics of nursing a baby with a cleft in the lip: if the palate is intact, the infant will be able to form a seal between the breast and the mouth and nose area, although the baby may nurse somewhat noisely (29). The mother's soft breast may mold to the open area between the mouth and nose, actually better than a firmer bottle nipple would (30). Some babies may have difficulty in maintaining a seal (31). The baby will have to undergo at least one corrective surgical procedure and will be hospitalized at those times. Following surgery and during the time of healing following each procedure, the baby may not be allowed to nurse, although some plastic surgeons now do allow such babies to resume nursings rapidly (32).
If the mother wants to resume nursing later, she will need to have expressed her milk each time breastfeeding was interrupted. Women who have continued nursing have felt that the effort was worthwhile because the nursings were emotionally satisfying for both mother and baby.

Cleft Palate

A baby born with one or more clefts in the palate or roof of the mouth may also either have an intact lip or one or more clefts in the lip. Normally in breastfeeding, a baby applies suction to the mother's nipple as he draws it up against the hard palate. Since a cleft in the palate prevents this, breastfeeding has been considered impossible. The baby theoretically is not able to maintain sufficient suction on the nipple to nurse. Yet in some cases breastfeeding has been possible. Much depends upon how extensive the cleft or clefts are. If the baby has only one cleft (unilateral cleft palate) and if this is fairly small and the rest of the palate is intact, the mother may be able to place her nipple in such a way that the cleft is avoided and the baby can nurse. How far out toward the gum the cleft extends is a consideration. A baby with two clefts or with one extensive cleft probably will not be able to nurse effectively.

The mother's emotional state and her interest in breastfeeding may have as much to do with her success at breastfeeding as the cleft itself. It has happened that a mother has nursed a baby with an undiagnosed small cleft palate quite successfully except that she noticed that milk ran out of the baby's nose if she lay down to nurse. Because the cleft was relatively small, and because the mother did not know that there was a problem, she went ahead and nursed. A mother who has been told that her baby has a birth defect may not want to become involved with an additional consideration, which breastfeeding may become in such cases. An emotional upset can make conditioning the let-down reflex more difficult. The decision to try to breastfeed is one that most mothers of cleft-palate babies do not make. The few who do want to nurse or express their milk can be advised of the experience of those who have done so successfully.

...... Suggestions For Nursing A Baby With A Cleft ......

1.   A mother whose baby has a small cleft in the palate may be able to nurse by holding the baby in an upright position.

2.   The woman should direct her nipple toward the part of the palate which is intact.

3.   The baby will find it easiest to drink the milk that is let down, and the mother may find it necessary to hand express milk directly into the baby's mouth after the initial let-down.

4.   The purpose of the suction (that is naturally maintained on the nipple by a baby with an intact palate) is to keep the nipple in position. Thus a woman may be able to compensate for the cleft palate by holding her nipple in the baby's mouth throughout the entire feeding, much as one holds a bottle nipple in an infant's mouth. One woman described her procedure:

> (The baby) could "milk" my breast, using her gums and tongue like I used my fingers. But because of the opening in the back of her mouth, when the tip of the nipple reached the cleft the suction would be broken and my nipple would drop back to the front of her mouth and out of it. The only purpose of suction, I realized, was to draw in and keep the nipple in her mouth.
>   I found that by placing my index finger on the top edge of the areola of my nipple and my middle finger on the bottom, I could press my nipple out between these fingers; it would protrude as if it were

full of milk. Andrea could now "milk" my nipple after I placed it in her mouth and empty my breast and fill herself up after the "let-down" had subsided (33).

5.   Babies have been fed breast milk in a bottle by mothers who have expressed their milk for weeks, sometimes months. The mothers must be enormously motivated and need support from those familiar with pumping and clefts.

6.   One idea that has been tried with disappointing results is the special cleft bottle nipple (duck bill shape). The rubber duck bill nipple is cut in half and the woman uses the top half as a breast shield to cover the baby's cleft palate. The problem is in getting a tight enough seal formed to keep the nipple in place to allow effective suckling.

7.   The Lact-Aid (Chapter 14) also has been tried, with mixed results. Women who are very motivated may be able to feed the baby at the breast in this way. In addition to motivation, the woman must have a nipple that is easy to grasp and a soft breast that will be able to be drawn into the baby's mouth and cover the open space in the palate. The mother may still need to help the baby maintain a hold on her nipple, so that it does not drop out of position in the baby's mouth.

It is clearly difficult to nurse a baby with a cleft palate and thus the suggestion to try should never come from an outsider, but from the mother who wants to nurse.

There are special support groups in the United States that provide inforation and support to families with cleft problems. The parents can be told that such groups exist and can be helped to find the nearest group.

CONTRAINDICATIONS TO BREASTFEEDING

Contraindications to nursing can be divided into baby-related and mother-related causes. The first group is mainly restricted to infants with inborn errors of metabolism such as galactosemia, phenylketonuria and maple syrup urine disease. In such cases special formulas which eliminate a particular substance are necessary.

Nursing may be difficult or impossible in the infant with extensive neurological defect sufficient to cause a poor suck and sometimes difficulty in swallowing. Such infants may even require nasogastric tube feeds.

Mother-related factors

Absolute contraindications to nursing include the necessity of long-term therapy of the mother with drugs which are unsafe to the nursing baby. (See Chapter 3)

Often cited is the mother with the communicable diseases, tuberculosis and pertussis, where close contact between mother and newborn is discouraged until the mother is no longer infectious. Pertussis however requires only 24 hours of erythromycin therapy to be given prior to allowing maternal-infant contact. Hopefully the diagnosis of active tuberculosis is made prior to term and treated appropriately. The woman whose tuberculosis is under control (that is, she is no longer infectious) can care for her own newborn; the safety of nursing is then limited by the medications that she requires. (See Chapter 3)

Excretion of viruses into breast milk has been documented (34, 35, 36, 37, 38) and in some cases may be of clinical significance. Although transmission of hepatitis from mother to newborn is believed most often to occur at the time of delivery, by oral or parenteral transmission, the possibility of transmission through breast milk is real (39). Women with active hepatitis at term, as well as women who are known hepatitis carriers, are probably best advised not to nurse. In the case of mild viral illnesses such as rubella, mumps, or other mild infections where transmission of disease to the infant causes little concern, there is no reason to interrupt nursing.

The practice of restricting the mother with a fever from nursing, or even from being with her baby during the postpartum period, needs re-evaluation. If the mother is not obviously "contagious" (as would be the case with untreated tuberculosis or whooping cough), and if she is well enough to want her baby, it is inappropriate to separate mother and infant.

A woman with severe psychological problems may be unable to care for or to nurse her own infant. Similarly, the severely retarded woman may require help in caring for her infant and nursing is likely to be difficult or impossible.

A very young mother, the thirteen or fourteen year old, needs considerable help in caring for her newborn (and may herself need most to return to school). Bottle feeding would ensure that the newborn's care can be a shared responsibility.

Complete absence of both breasts and/or nipples is a very rare anomaly which makes lactation impossible (40).

MANAGEMENT OF DRUG THERAPY FOR LACTATING WOMEN

A lactating woman whose condition requires drug therapy often is able to continue nursing. It is appropriate for the physician who prescribes any medication to a nursing mother to be aware of possible effects on the baby, to limit the use of medications to only those absolutely required, and to select the safest ones when a choice is possible (e.g. another antibiotic can almost always be substituted for tetracycline).

With the exception of relatively few drugs (Chapter 3), most drugs are considered safe for the lactating woman.

On occasion, a mother who requires long-term therapy, often with multiple drugs which are believed to be individually safe, notices that her infant is suffering an undesirable effect—such as the child of an asthmatic on multiple medications being tremulous. If the effect seems to be consistent and real, and if the medications are needed on a long-term basis, a trial of formula-feeds may be advised, while mother pumps her breasts. If the child clearly improves, it is advisable to suggest weaning. Also, that the infant will not nurse for several hours after a maternal dose of a medication may be difficult to predict, especially in the very young infant who nurses frequently. These factors, as well as peculiarities of metabolism of the drug within an infant may influence what drug effect can be expected.

References

1. Gartner, L: Severe or prolonged unconjugated hyperbilirubemia of the newborn, in Rudolph, AM, ed., *Pediatrics.* New York: Appleton-Century Crofts, 1977.

2. Arias, O, Gartner, L, et al.: Prolonged neonatal unconjugated hyperbilirubinemia associated with breastfeeding and a steroid pregnane 3 (α) 20 (βdiol) diet, J. Clin. Invest. 43:2037, 1964.

3. Arthur, et al.: Breast milk conjugation inibitors, Arch. Dis. Child. 47:987, 1972.

4. Cole, Hargreaves: Conjugation inhibitions and early neonatal hyperbilirubinemia. Arch. Dis Child. 47:415, 1972.

. Gartner, L: Unconjugated neonatal hyperbilirubemia, in Rudolph, AM, ed., *Pediatrics.* New York: Appleton-Century Crofts, 1977.

. Arias, O, et al.: Transient familial neonatal hyperbilirubenemia. J. Clin. Invest. 44:1442, 1965.

. Applebaum, RM: Breast feeding and care of the breasts, from Davis' *Gynecology and Obstetrics, I.* Chapter 32, Hagerstown. Maryland: Harper and Row, Inc., 1974.

. Rice, I: *Heartstart: A practical guide to breast-feeding.* St. Paul: Ilene Rice, 2392 Nancy Place, St. Paul, MN, 1977.

. American Academy of Pediatrics Committee on Nutrition: Commentary on Breast-Feeding, Pediatr. 62:59, 1978.

10. Heird, WC and Anderson, TL: Nutritional requirements and methods of feeding low birth weight infants. Curr. Probl. Pediatr. vii: June, 1977.

11. Gordon, HH, Levine, SJ, McNamana, H: Feeding of the premature infant a combination of human and cow's milk, Anal. Child. Dis. 73: 442, 1947.

12. Heird, WC: Feeding the Premature infant, Am. J. Dis. Child. 131:468, 1977.

13. Kagan, BM, Felix, N et al: Body water changes in relation to nutrition of premature infants. Ann. N.Y. Acad. Sci. 110:830, 1963.

14. Davies, DP: Adequacy of expressed milk for early growth of preterm infants, Arch. Dis. Child. 52:296, 1977.

15. Fomon, SJ et al: Human milk and the small premature infant, Am. J. Dis. Child. 131: 464, 1977.

16. Raiha, NCR et al: Milk protein quantity and quality in low-birth-weight infants: 1. Metabolic responses and effects on growth, Pediatrics 57:659, 1976.

17. Rassin, DK et al.: Milk protein quantity and quality in low-birth-weight infants. IV. Effects on tyrosure and phenylanine in plasma and urine. J. Pediatr. 90:356, 1977.

18. Rassin, DK et al: Milk protein. II. Effects on selected aliphatic amino acids in plasma and urine, Pediatrics 59:407, 1977.

19. Gaull, GE et al. Milk protein quantity to quality in low-birth-weight infants. III. Effects on sulfur amino acids in plasma and urine, J. Pediatr. 90:348, 1977.

20. Atkinson et al: Human milk: differences in nitrogen concentration in milk from mothers of term and premature infants, J. Pediatr. 93: 67, 1978.

21. Pitt, J et al: Protection against experimental necrotizing enterocolitis by maternal milk, Pediatr. Res. 11:906, 1977.

22. Addy, HA: The breast-feeding of twins, Environmental child health 231, 1975.

23. La Leche League International: I Just Took It for Granted (Reprint No. 54 Twins), June, 1971.

24. Breastfeeding Your Twins. Willow Grove, PA: Health Education Associates, 1978.

25. Trainham, G, et al: A case history of twins breast fed on a self-demand regime, J. Pediatr. 27:97, 1954.

26. Klaus, M and Kennell, J: *Maternal-infant bonding.* St. Louis: The C.V. Mosby Company, 1976.

27. Auerback, KG, coordinator: Breastfeeding the Premature Infant. Keeping Abreast Journal II:98, 1977.

28. Nursing the Down's Syndrome Baby. Franklin Park, Illinois, LLLI.

29. Beck, F: Breastfeeding the baby with a cleft lip, Keeping Abreast J. of Human Nurturing III:122, 1978.

30. Smale, S: Nursing a Baby with Cleft Lip. The CEA Philadelphia Chronicler II (7), 1975.

31. Wealterly, White, RCA: Breastfeeding the baby with a cleft lip, Keeping Abreast, Journal of Human Nurturing III (2), 1978, p. 125.

32. Graham, William P., Professor of Surgery, Chief of Plastic Surgery, Milton S. Hershey Medical Center, Penn State University, Hershey, Pennsylvania (Interview).

33. Grady, E: Breastfeeding the baby with a cleft of the soft palate, Keeping Abreast, J. of Human Nurturing III (2), 1978, p. 126.

34. Lunnemann, CC and Goldberg, S: Hepatitis B Antigen in breast milk, Lancet 2:155, 1974.

35. Baxall, EH, Flewett, TH, et al. Hepatitis B surface antigen in breast milk, Lancet 2:1007-8, 1974.

36. Hayes, K: Cytmegalosurus in Human Milk, New Engl. J. Med. 287:177, 1972.

37. Burmovici, Klein, Elena, et al: Isolation of rubella virus in milk after postpartum immunization. J. Pediatr. 91:940, 1977.

38. Dunkle, LM, et al: Neonatal herpes simplex infection possibly acquired via maternal breast milk, Pediatrics 63:250, 1979.

39. Crunpack, CS: Hepatitis in infectious diseases of the fetus and newborn infant, Remington, JS and Klein, JO, eds., Philadelphia: W.B Sanders, 1976, p. 492.

40. Haagensen, CD: *Diseases of the Breast.* Philadelphia, W.B. Saunders Company, 1971.

Chapter 8

Breast Problems

GENERAL DISCUSSION

A number of common problems can be causes of lactation failure. Soreness or nipple pain and engorgement may cause woman to wean (1,2,3,4) often before lactation is established. Problems in conditioning the let-down reflex ultimately may cause failure at breastfeeding (5,6,7,8). Some women have reported that they abandoned breastfeeding because they found leaking breasts to be so offensive. Mastitis or breast abscess also may cause women to wean (9). Proper handling and avoidance of these common problems are, therefore, vital in attaining and then maintaining optimal lactation.

The problems need not occur as often as they do at present (10); preventing or minimizing them before they occur is feasibile (11).

There are two recommended practices that are effective in preventing or minimizing all of the above problems. These two practices are frequent nursings and varying the nursing position.

Frequent nursings with the use of both breasts at each feeding is universally valuable advice for all new breastfeeding mothers. The nursings should initially be held to a maximum of 5 to 10 minutes on each breast. The length of each nursing should be extended gradually, as long as the nipple/areola skin remains healthy and comfortable. If the mother's nipples are becoming sore or fissured, the length of each nursing should be shortened. The baby will continue to receive adequate amounts of milk as most of the milk is obtained in the first 5-10 minutes of nursing (when let-down occurs promptly). There is clinical experience that initial feedings many times are too long. Many women who have followed a plan of prolonged nursings in the beginning (for as long as the baby wants) (11) have indeed become sore. A vigorous newborn may suckle for 45 minutes or more for many feedings day and night. These women report that the nipple soreness not only appeared sooner, as was expected, but also was more severe than with previous nursing experiences in which their initial feedings were held to 10 minutes on each breast (and later feedings gradually lengthened).

Frequent, short nursings also prevent other problems. Engorgement is prevented when milk is removed regularly (12). Problems with plugged ducts are avoided because, when milk is removed regularly, stasis is prevented.

The other piece of advice, to vary the nursing positions, is of secondary importance to the necessity for frequent nursings—but it is still valuable for new mothers. Variation is accomplished by sitting up for some feedings and lying down for others. This helps prevent soreness by varying the points of greatest stress on the nipple and the areola skin.

Women who report that they are able to nurse in only one position may not have made an effort to learn an alternative position. As long as they do not develop a problem with soreness or cracking in one particular area of the nipple, they need not be urged to modify their preference for one position. However, women to whom the value of varying the nursing position as a preventive measure against soreness and cracking is explained, generally master two or more positions with no difficulty.

Varying the nursing positions minimizes problems with plugged ducts because the strongest nursing action, near the infant's chin, is moved to different points around the breast.

Women who are advised to use frequent, but initially short, nursings and to vary the nursing positions thus are able to avoid or minimize common problems; and prevention is far easier than cure.

It is not uncommon for a new mother to have problems simultaneously. Soreness and engorgement often are found together. An inhibited let-down, leading to engorgement, is common early on in new mothers. Often one problem directly causes another problem. The inhibited let-down causes engorgement, as milk is being made but is not being removed by the baby. This in turn can cause nipple soreness: when the milk does not let down, the hungry infant chews frantically at the nipple and this can cause nipple and areola damage.

Once a problem occurs, it is useful to review her nursing routine with the new mother. Often a "nursing indiscretion" or error can be found in a mother who complains of sore nipples, engorgement or other problems. To summarize, some common nursing indiscretions are nursing too long in the first week, failing to use both breasts at most feedings, nursing with the infant's mouth on just the tip of the mother's nipple, and failing to nurse frequently during the times when the baby is most alert.

In order to help a woman with a particular breast problem, then, it i necessary to discover any nursing indiscretions. Telling a woman who complains of sore nipples, for example, that she should air-dry her nipples or use a heat lamp or use a breast-care cream are common recommendations. Yet these recommendations will be inadequate if the woman continues prolonged nursing on one breast at a time. A hot shower is an inadequate recommendation for engorgement if the woman continues to go too long between nursings.

PROBLEMS WITH NIPPLE PROTRACTILITY

Most problems with non-graspable nipples can be prevented, or at least minimized, with appropriate prenatal and postpartum management (13). See Chapter 5 for a discussion of nipple types and remedies for non-graspable nipples. It is important to remember that the two main corrective measures [the Hoffman Technique (14,15,16,17) and the use of a milk cup], (18,19) which should ideally be carried out prenatally, are also effective when done postpartum.

Figure 8-1 demonstrates the importance of nipple protractility. In nursing, the infant draws the nipple and areola into his mouth. He then draws the nipple up against the hard palate. His tongue is in the front of his mouth and strokes the bottom of the mother's nipple (16).

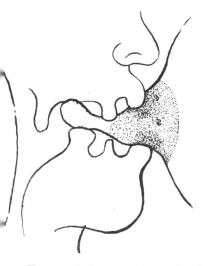

Figure 8-1. Protractile nipple drawn into infant's mouth (exaggerated schematic drawing).

Two points can be made from this illustration: 1. The infant does not obtain milk from "sucking" on the nipple, as one sucks with a straw. The infant's mouth must be well back on the areola in order to compress the lacteal sinuses, where the milk is stored. These lacteal sinuses lie 1-1½ inches back from the nipple. The milking action then is not sucking but rather compressing. The infant's tongue strokes the milk out. 2. Effective nipple preparation is mandatory for the woman with non-protractile nipples; otherwise the infant is likely to be unable to draw the nipple back into his mouth and breastfeeding fails.

There are reports of success in drawing out problem nipples by using the suction created by electric (20) or hand pumps, both before and after the baby is born. One report suggested using a plastic and rubber nipple shield. The rubber end of the shield is cut away. The remaining plastic of the shield is placed over the areola and suction is applied with a hand pump (21).

It is rare to find a nipple that is completely inverted all the way around. More often the nipple inverts on one side but comes out on the other side, the so-called semi-inverted nipple. Sometimes a nipple continues to invert between feedings in spite of prenatal nipple preparation and nursing.

Findings of Women
. . . . Who Have Nursed with Inverted Nipples . . . .

1.   Babies prefer the regular nipple if only one inverts, but can be coaxed to nurse on the inverted side and are sometimes able to draw the nipple out. The mother must be patient and persistent to coax her baby to keep trying. Some women find this to be too much trouble and switch to bottle feeding.

2.   An inverted or flat nipple is more likely to become sore and even cracked. The mother should be urged to alternate nursing positions, air dry after feedings, etc.

3.   Very rarely, a woman with one very inverted nipple finds that her baby continues to be frustrated and cannot seem to nurse on the problem side. Women have nursed successfully on just one side.

Summary of Measures for Preventing
. . . . Problems with Nipple Graspability. . . . .

1.   Appropriate prenatal preparation should be given to problem nipples.

2.   After delivery, frequent nursings around the clock should be given to prevent engorgement, which makes any nipple appear flat and be difficult to grasp.

3.   The infant is half the nursing team. Minimal medication in labor and delivery will help to enable the infant to nurse

vigorously (22). The infant should be brought to the mother for nursings when he is alert; rooming-in is ideal.

When prenatal treatment was not carried out or was not completely successful, the following points can be made to the woman:

Postpartum Treatment for Managing
. . . . .Non-Graspable Nipples . . . .

1.   Use ice (crushed ice in a clean cloth) or a cold cloth plus hand shaping to try to form a flat nipple.

2.   Use the Hoffman Technique and wear a milk cup between and just before nursings to help train the nipple to stand out.

3.   Use a nipple shield (pre-moistened for proper contact). Instruct each mother in the correct use of a shield, that is, *used only at the beginning of the nursings* to draw the nipple out. Then remove the shield and put the baby back onto the mother's formed nipple (23). (For more on shields, see Chapter 14)

ENGORGEMENT

Engorgement refers to overfullness in the breasts. All new mothers have some degree of fullness, but not all become engorged. In all new mothers, with the onset of lactation the breasts become larger, heavier and tender. This is normal and is due not only to the production of milk, but also to increased lymph and blood supply to the breasts (24).

If a new mother does not nurse frequently enough, the normal fullness of early lactation is likely to develop into massive congestion, as milk is made but is not removed (17,25). With engorgement, the breasts are hard, painful and warm to the touch. The skin looks shiney. The nipple appears flat because of the overfullness of the breast. It is difficult or impossible for the baby to draw the nipple and areolar skin into his mouth.

. . . .Solutions for Preventing or Managing Engorgement . . . .

1.   Scheduling frequent, but initially short, nursings day and night is the most important preventive measure. In a hospital with no option except the traditional four-hour schedule, the mother can be advised to nurse twice, at the beginning and then at the end of each session with the infant.

2.   The woman can wear a milk cup before a feeding to encourage her nipple to stand out. She can also wear the cup on the other side while nursing from the first breast. This will help to hold that second nipple out from the fullness of the breast.

3.   She can hand-express a small amount of milk before a feeding in order to soften the area behind the nipple and thus make the nipple easier for the infant to grasp. This should be done gently.

4.   This hand-expression can be preceded by a warm or comfortably hot shower. The woman should be advised to stand with her back to the water and let the water run over her shoulders towards her breasts.

5.   The woman can be advised to do relaxation breathing or take some slow deep breaths to help get her let-down going.

6.   The woman can use warm packs to relax the tissues before a feeding, and cold packs after a feeding, if needed, for comfort and to reduce swelling. The use of heat is more widely accepted than is the use of cold. It has been suggested that ice is effective in reducing swelling, although the practice has been questioned by some.

The extra fullness within the breasts subsides without treatment within a week, or two after delivery. All new mothers need to be forewarned about this: the swelling (not the milk) will go away. Women often fear that they have lost their milk when this occurs.

LEAKING

Not all women leak. Many do, to varying degrees. A woman nursing for the second time may notice that she has less leaking. Fortunately this is not because she has less milk the second time.

The woman who does not leak at all may need reassurance of the adequacy of her milk supply while women who do leak may need to be reassured that it is normal. Although leaking decreases or stops in many women with time, some women continue to leak over many months of nursing, some through the entire period of lactation.

To stop the flow of milk temporarily, the woman can press the heel of her hand to the nipple through her clothing or cross her arms inconspicuously across her chest and apply firm pressure. At the beginning of feeding, many women need to exert pressure against the other breast as they milk lets-down simultaneously in both breasts.

Other Suggestions

Advise the mother to use bra pads without a plastic liner, except perhaps on special occasions. The plastic cuts off contact with the air and can cause sore nipples.

For a woman who is bothered by leaking heavily from the other side while nursing, recommend that she wear a milk cup (see Chapter 14) during the feeding. If there is proper sterilizing, and attention is paid to getting the milk refrigerated very quickly, the milk may be saved. If a woman wears the cup between feedings, the milk collected by dripping in must be discarded. Wearing the cups continually to collect leaking milk is not recommended. The constant gentle pressure on the sinuses will actually stimulate more leaking.

Leaking can happen when the woman thinks about her baby and her let-down is triggered (7).

Leaking during sexual intercourse is very common. (Oxytocin is released during orgasm.) Leaking can be decreased by advising the woman to nurse prior to intercourse so that the breasts are relatively empty. She may need to be reassured that this leaking is a normal thing.

SORENESS

Sore nipples may be the most common complaint of breastfeeding women. The term "sore nipples" may be used to describe sensations ranging from a slight discomfort of the nipple and areola skin at the onset of a feeding to excruciating pain when the nipples are cracked and tender. The term "soreness" then is used to describe many breast conditions.

Soreness that occurs when an infant is first placed at the breast in the 1-3 minute period before the milk begins to flow (lets-down) is normal. This time at the beginning of each nursing is often described as uncomfortable and may represent "suction unrelieved by swallowing" (2) (the baby sucking without swallowing before the milk begins to flow). The pain disappears as the milk lets-down and the infant begins to swallow. No treatment is indicated unless the discomfort is great. In cases of great discomfort, the mother may wish to try to trigger a let-down through breast massage before putting the baby onto the breast. A strong tingling sensation which begins 1-2 minutes into nursing and then fades may be the let-down reflex. Again, this most often is not a severe pain and needs no treatment. Mothers may wonder, however, whether it is normal and they can be reassured.

Often, however, sore nipples follow incorrect technique and represent true damage to the nipple and areola skin. Nursing too long initially, nursing without prompt let-down (mother inexperienced, frightened, embarrassed), incorrect positioning of the areola in baby's mouth, the improper use of breast shields, and improper care of the nipples are possible causes. Table 8-1 lists the causes and cures.

Causes and Cures of Nipple Soreness—A Summary

There are, then, a number of measures that can be taken to alleviate nipple soreness. Some of them can be classified as general "comfort measures." These are particularly useful to the mother of a newborn, the mother whose nipple/areola skin is not yet accustomed to nursing. However, these comfort measures for "normal newborn soreness" are useful also for the mother of an older baby where soreness may be due to other causes.

. . . . .Comfort Measures for Soreness . . . .

1.　Rotate positions.

2.　Give short, frequent nursings.

3.　Practice relaxation techniques at the beginning of feeding.

4.　Nurse on the less sore side first.

5.　Make sure baby's mouth is well back on the areola.

6.　Be sure that baby is removed properly from the breast, breaking suction.

7.　Air dry after each feeding. The use of an ultraviolet ray sunlamp or bulb (for 30 seconds, increasing over time to 60 or 90 seconds) has been recommended; however reports of women burning themselves are not uncommon. Air drying and/or sunlight work well and are safer.

8.　Use *small* amounts of breast-care cream, being careful not to clog the nipple pores and using always after air-drying. A cream such as Eucerin may be indicated for very dry skin, but appears to have only a placebo effect on soreness.

9.　Possibly use ice to numb a sore nipple.

The following table summarizes many of the causes of nipple soreness and possible solutions.

Table 8-1
Nipple Soreness: Causes and Solutions

Possible Cause	Solutions
1. Nipple/areola skin not yet accustomed to nursing.	Use comfort measures (above)
2. Baby very hard on nipples, possible indication that mother is stalling feedings (making the baby wait 3 or 4 hours between feedings). The baby is hard on the nipples because he is very hungry. Stalling feedings also contributes to engorgement, which stretches the skin and makes nursing difficult.	Nurse on demand.
3. Nursing too long, more than 10 minutes per breast before nipples are accustomed to nursing.	Keep each feeding to approximately 10 minutes, shorter time if very sore, lengthening as soreness disappears.
4. Poorly protractile nipples (flat, inverted, engorged)	(a) Give short, frequent nursings to prevent engorgement. (b) Use ice before the feeding to make a reluctant nipple become erect. (c) Use milk cup before feedings, Hoffman technique between feedings. (d) Use nipple shield only at beginning of nursing. (e) Use comfort measures.
5. Wearing a rubber breast shield or a plastic and rubber nipple shield for the duration of the feeding. These rub, making skin sore, and can prevent let-down, leading to engorgement. Five minutes without a shield accomplishes much more than 20 minutes with.	Avoid shields for all uses except drawing out non-protractile nipples. For that use, remove shield within two minutes.
6. Irritation of nipples by chemicals. The use of irritants may not be immediately apparent. They might be drying agents such as soap, alcohol, Wash 'n' Dry, other germ-killing preparations, shampoo running over breasts in the shower, and spray deodorant.	(a) Avoid all suspect chemicals (b) Use comfort measures.

7. Bra pad or bra flap may stick to nipple/areola skin, if the mother leaks. They even may remove a small amount of skin when the mother pulls the bra flap open.	(a) Use cloth bra pads. (b) If a commercial bra pad or bra flap is stuck, moisten it with water before opening the bra.
8. Occluding air from the nipples. This may be caused by failing to air dry, using a plastic-lined bra, or wearing a milk cup between feedings for the purpose of keeping clothes dry.	(a) Air dry. (b) Use appropriate bra pads, or cotton handkerchiefs. (c) Avoid wearing milk cup routinely.
9. Mother is not letting-down. Baby is sucking vigorously although no milk is available.	Help the mother to relax and nurse on demand in comfortable surroundings. Massage breast. Possibly use Syntocinon. (See page 138)

Soreness problems that often occur after the early weeks

10. Thrush (Check baby's mouth for white patches, in cases of *persistent* soreness.)	(a) Use Nystatin, 100,000 units/cc; 1 cc four times a day orally. (b) Gentian violet (aqueous) as a second choice to Nystatin. (c) Use comfort measures.

Older baby/toddler soreness problems

11. Teething. Some teething babies tend to use a chewing mouth action. Some mothers feel that the saliva of the older teething baby is irritating.	(a) Keep the nursings fairly short. End the feeding if the older baby changes from a sucking mouth action to a chewing action. (b) The mother may want to wash her breasts with warm water after each nursing. (c) Use comfort measures.
12. Biting	(a) Saying "no" firmly and ending the nursing without screaming. (b) Watch for a change in the sucking pattern and be ready to end the feeding. (c) Watch for a playful look on baby's face. (d) Keep finger at corner of baby's mouth, ready to break suction. (e) Avoid "snack" nursings (numerous, very brief nursings).
13. Increased (more frequent and/or longer) nursings, often due to illness, teething, separation anxiety, and growth spurts.	(a) Try to determine reason for increased nursings, if unknown. (b) Use comfort measures.

14. Toddler with food or foreign matter in his mouth.	Check toddler's mouth before nursings for cookie crumbs, sand, etc.
15, Undiagnosed early pregnancy is another explanation for mysteriously sore nipples in women with older babies.	(a) Use comfort measures. (b) Shorten nursings. (c) Decision on weaning.

In nursing, the baby's mouth flattens or compresses the nipple and areolar skin between his gums. There is a compression line between the part of the mother's breast in the baby's mouth and the rest of the breast. The compression line, then, is the line formed across the breast from corner to corner of the baby's mouth. The points compressed, the points at the two corners of the baby's mouth, receive greater stress than the rest of the nipple and areola, and so are most apt to become sore. The part of the nipple/areola that is stroked by the baby's tongue also receives greater stress and so is more apt to become sore (2). So there are three points receiving greater than average stress. Varying the nursing position (sitting, lying, football hold) then will allow a sore nipple/areola to heal while the baby is continuing to nurse (see Chapter 7).

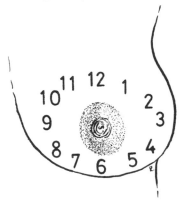

Figure 8-2. Clock positions.

Describing the breast as the face of a clock is helpful in communicating with a woman about the points of stress over the telephone (see Fig. 8-2). "You say that your nipple is really sore. Let's think of your breast as a face of a clock, with twelve at the top, six o'clock at the bottom of your breast, nearest to your waist. Where is the sorest spot?" A woman whose soreness is worse at a certain part of the nipple/areola skin (at seven o'clock, for example) can most benefit from changing the nursing position. In addition to the common positions, sitting up, lying down, football hold, consider suggesting that the woman lie down and place the baby lying on his side with his legs extending away from the mother's shoulders (see Fig. 8-3). This can seem awkward but has the advantage of putting the three stress points at locations different from the common ones. It may be indicated to avoid a crack on the lower part of the nipple, where most cracks occur. Women with cracked nipples are grateful to be told of the position.

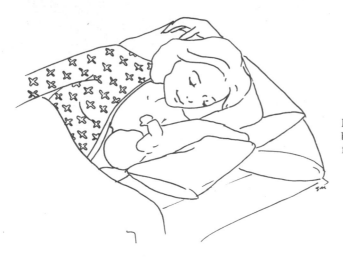

Figure 8-3. Nursing with baby's legs extending away from mother's shoulder.

A woman who complains of soreness may be offered a breast-care cream. A cream is indicated to cure dryness and ease soreness, but it is not a cure-all and is contraindicated if the skin is macerated. Pure hydrous lanolin has been recommended (3), but may cause a reaction in a woman allergic to wool products.

Brand-name breast care creams are available but contain multiple ingredients. Eucerin cream is a pure cream and hydrating agent and can be used for women with dry skin (17).

In a controlled study the use of creams was found to have a placebo effect (mothers felt they were doing something for the problem) but there was no objective effect (3).

Fissured or Cracked Nipples
Sore nipples sometimes develop into fissured or cracked nipples (2). Fissures are usually found on the under side of the nipple, since the commonly used nursing positions place more stress on this area.

...... Suggestions to Help Cure the Fissured Nipple ......

1.   Discuss the mother's nursing routines with her to discover and eliminate any nursing errors.

2.   Recommend that the mother use a nursing position that places the points of stress away from the fissure. (See earlier this chapter)

3.   Recommend comfort measures, especially having the woman begin each feeding on the breast without the fissure.

4. Encourage the woman to try to get the infant's mouth even farther up on the areola to avoid the fissure. She can compress her breast with the scissor hold.

5. The use of a mild analgesic may be indicated.

6. Encourage the mother to continue with short, frequent nursings. If nursings are infrequent, the resulting engorgements would stretch the skin.

Note: Mothers may become alarmed at the darkening of the infant's stools, which may occur secondary to absorbed blood from a bleeding nipple.

Blisters

Blisters on the tip of the nipple occur occasionally and may be filled with clear fluid or blood. The mother should be advised to let the blister open naturally; they heal spontaneously.

. . . . . Suggestions for Nursing When There is a Blister. . . . . .

1. Start nursing on the other, good side.

2. Help the mother to find a nursing position in which the points of the compression line and the tongue stroking do not hit the blister.

3. Keep the nursings brief.

4. Advise the woman to soak with warm compresses before nursing.

PROBLEMS WITH THE LET-DOWN REFLEX

The let-down reflex (the milk ejection reflex, or the draught reflex) is normally conditioned during the early weeks of nursing. The let-down reflex takes a variable time to be conditioned and may not be fully conditioned for several weeks in the first-time nurser (7). The mother who is not bothered by sore nipples should increase the duration of her nursings in order to provide the needed stimulation. The mother who does have sore nipples, but who still needs to condition her let-down reflex, may wish to use breast massage before nursing in order to help trigger the reflex. If the reflex can be triggered before the infant is placed at the breast, the time that he is at the breast before the milk flows is shortened.

With a conditioned let-down, the infant's suckling promptly triggers the release of oxytocin. The milk begins to flow within seconds and may spray from the nipple pores in streams. Without the let-down reflex, the milk which has been produced cannot be delivered to the hungry infant; the infant is able to obtain only the small amount of watery foremilk.

The fact that the let-down can be triggered by the mother's thinking about the infant or hearing the infant cry suggests the importance of psychological factors. Many factors, such as pain, fear or embarrassment, may inhibit this reflex.

Although problems with the let-down can be largely prevented, when they do occur, they are often the most difficult situations in breastfeeding management to treat.

. . . . .Signs of a Functioning Let-Down . . . .

1.   Multiparas, especially, notice uterine contractions during nursing in the early postpartum period. Increased vaginal bleeding also may be noted. These signs are noted most strongly in a woman who has nursed previously. Her let-down reflex, already conditioned during nursing the previous infant, can be expected to function sooner than would that of a woman nursing for the first time, even if she is a multipara.

2.   Some women notice a sensation of tingling, or fullness in the breast, a "kind of a pain."

3.   Leaking from the unsuckled breast while nursing is also evidence of a functioning let-down.

4.   A change in the infant's suckling pattern is an important clue, especially in women who have not noticed other signs of a let-down. A change in the infant's swallowing pattern, which may be accompanied by a gulping sound, indicates that the baby is getting milk. This sign is more consistent than any of the other signs.

5.   Some women notice a feeling of well-being or relaxation at let-down, somewhat similar to the feelings that follow orgasm. Some women describe an intense thirst; rarely a woman experiences orgasm with each let-down. Although some of these women enjoy this phenomenon, others are repelled and worried by it and want to wean.

Preventing Problems with the Let-Down Reflex

The most effective way to prevent problems with the let-down reflex is to provide a source of encouragement and emotional support to the new mother, in order that she be as relaxed as possible in the postpartum period. Mother and baby can be kept together as much as possible, and frequent feeds can be encouraged, as soon as the baby awakens and before he is crying angrily with hunger. Hospital stays that encourage confidence in the mother's own ability to care for her infant also help to produce relaxed mothers.

Because conditioned stimulation can produce the let-down reflex, the use of routines is beneficial to the woman with a let-down problem, as well as for any woman who is conditioning her let-down:

. . . . Suggestions for Conditioning the Let-Down Reflex . . . .

1.   Encourage her to nurse in a place that is quiet and free from annoyances and to be in a comfortable nursing position.

2.   Suggest that the woman do relaxation breathing (exercises taught in classes in prepared childbirth), or take a few deep breaths before each nursing. If it helps her to relax, she can watch TV, listen to music, or she may want to and can be encouraged to pick up the baby and just watch and hold him for awhile, nursing every 2-2½ hours during the day.

3.   Suggest that the woman drink something just before every nursing (tea, juice, water, an occasional beer or glass of wine).

4.   If leaking occurs, the mother can pick up the baby and nurse, if it is close to two hours since the last feeding.

5.   Encourage women to rest adequately during the first days and weeks at home.

Following are some indications that there may be more serious difficulties:

Clues that there may be a Problem
. . . . with the Let-Down Reflex. . . . .

1.   The woman has *none* of the let-down signs.

2.   The baby wants to nurse constantly and never is content.

3.   There is low weight gain.

4.   The mother says that the nighttime feedings go better than those in the day time; the baby sleeps after those feedings. Nervous mothers seem to relax better when they are alone or sleepy.

5.   The mother seems unusually nervous and says that she doesn't relax when she nurses.

For a Persistent Let-Down Problem

These problems are not easy to work with. Sometimes the woman may not want to forget clocks and schedules and just nurse. She may prefer instead to forego nursing altogether, finding that the needed relaxed life style which revolves around the newborn is not for her. In addition to the suggestions already given on preventing problems with the let-down reflex, breast massage or synthetic oxytocin (Syntocinon), administered in a nasal spray, may be useful in some cases. (One or two sprays into a nostril prior to nursing. It must be used several times during a feeding.) Oxytocin may be useful for women with persistent let-down problems as well as for women trying to let-down to a breast pump, who truly want to nurse. (Syntocinon is available in the United States but the pharmacy may need to place a special order for the medication since it is not widely prescribed.) The use of this medication is not a cure-all for let-down problems. Some women find it objectionable becuase of associated painful sensations (head pain, too strong a let-down). Some women have a deep-seated, although often hidden, aversion to nursing, which may present as a let-down problem. These women will not be helped by oxytocin nasal nor by prescribing chloropromozine. Often they have chosen to nurse because of peer or other outside pressure.

PLUGGED DUCTS

Sometimes a mother describes a local area of tenderness and a palpable tiny lump within the tender area. There appear to be local accumulations of milk or dead cells that have been shed and cause a blockage in the duct and may be called plugged or clogged ducts. "Caked breast" refers to this same process occurring in a larger area of a breast (multiple plugged ducts).

Plugged ducts may be caused by external pressure, such as a tight bra or bunched nightclothes under the arm, both of which prohibit satisfactory emptying of the breast. Another contributing factor is stasis, going too long between feedings.

Plugged ducts may be very frightening to a woman who connects a breast lump with breast cancer. The movement of a plug down a duct and its eventual disappearance clearly differentiates this condition from cancer.

...... Suggestions for Dealing with a Plugged Duct.......

1.   Nurse more frequently, always starting with the affected breast.

2.   Change the nursing position so that the baby's chin is positioned closest to the sore spot, for the strongest sucking action.

3.   While nursing on the affected side, the woman may use the warm heat of a wet cloth and *gently* massage to encourage proper drainage and help move the plug down the duct.

4.   Between nursings, the mother may use moist heat and gentle manual manipulation to encourage the lump to travel down the duct. She also may use gentle massage in the shower or tub, or with the breast submerged in a clean basin of warm water.

5.   The mother should try to remove any dried secretion that may be blocking nipple pores. She should avoid putting nipple cream over the nipple pores.

6.   She should get extra rest and good diet, a properly fitting bra, avoid omitting nursings.

SPORADIC NON-EPIDEMIC MASTITIS (BREAST INFECTION)

Mastitis is a soft-tissue infection of the breast, most often caused by staphylococcus aureus in the setting of milk stasis. It can predispose to breast abscess, if it is not treated properly.

...............Symptoms of Infection...............

1.   Fever

2.   Redness; breast is tender to the touch.

3.   Generalized aching

"Flu" in a nursing mother should be regarded as a breast infection until proven otherwise.

...... Times When Mastitis is Most Likely to Occur. ......

1.   During the newborn period, especially when the breast is not emptied properly or when the mother is especially tired.

2.   Following abrupt weaning.

3.   Any time there is a large variation in supply and demand.

4.   When the mother is nursing twins.

The mother with mastitis should be encouraged to keep nursing (26,27) to prevent stasis: breast abscess is most likely to develop if nursing is abruptly stopped. If continued nursing is not possible (for instance, if the child is recently weaned or too ill), the milk must be removed from the breasts with an effective breast pump, or by hand expression. Avoidance of stasis is crucial.

.... The Treatment of Mastitis is as Follows. ....

1.   Heat—warm, moist compresses, or a baby's hot water bottle. Heating pads sometimes are associated with skin burns.

2.   Rest –Tell the woman to go directly to bed.

3.   Empty breast—The mother should nurse frequently, keeping the baby's chin close to the sore area. This may help keep area well drained. Start nursing on the affected side and keep that breast empty.

4.   Antibiotics—Although the infection can often be handled with the above measures, mastitis is a potentially serious infection and anit-staphylococcal oral antibiotics are indicated (dicloxicillin [125 mg-250 mg q6h] or an oral cephalosporin [250 mg cephalexin q6h] in penicillin allergic women). If antibiotics are not started initially, the woman must be watched carefully—and if symptoms persist 24 hours, antibiotics should then definitely be started.

Montgomery Glands Can Get Infected Too

An infection of the Montgomery glands is a more superficial infection. It can be treated locally with moist heat. Often these infections are associated with misuse of creams. Nursing can be continued, but a different nursing position may be necessary to avoid stress on the sore area.

BREAST ABSCESS

Breast abscess is found most often following sudden weaning in the face of mastitis. It requires surgical drainage and is often extremely painful. Nursing is usually not possible from the involved breast. This is a serious infection, best avoided by prompt vigorous treatment of mastitis with continued frequent nursing.

References

1. Waller, H: The early failure of breast feeding. A clinical study of its causes and their prevention, Arch. Dis. Child. 21:1, 1946.

2. Gunther, M: Sore nipples, causes and prevention, Lancet 2:590, 1945.

3. Newton, M: Nipple pain and nipple damage: problems in management of breast feeding, J. Pediatr. 41:411, 1952.

4. Newton, M: Postpartum engorgement of the breast, Am. J. Obstet. Gynecol. 61:664, 1951.

5. Newton, M and Egli, GE: The effect of intranasal administration of oxytocin on the let-down of milk in lactating women, Am. J. Obstet. Gynecol. 76:103, 1958.

6. Raphael, D: *The Tender Gift: Breastfeeding.* Englewood Cliffs, New Hersey: Prentice Hall, 1973.

7. Isbister, C: A clinical study of the draught reflex in human lactation, Arch. Dis. Child 29: 143, 1954.

8. Newton, M and Newton, N: The let-down reflex in human lactation, J. Pediatr. 3:698, 1948.

9. Newton, M: Breast abscess: a result of lactation failure, Surgery, Gynecol. Obstet. 91: 651, 1950.

10. Applebaum, RM: The physician and a common sense approach to breast feeding, Sout. Med. J. 63:793, 1970.

11. Haire, D: The nurse's contribution to successful breast-feeding and the medical value of breast-feeding. Chapter V of *Implementing Family Centered Maternity Care.* International Childbirth Education Association, 1974.

12. Applebaum, RM: The obstetrician's approach to the breasts and breast-feeding, J. Reprod. Med. 14:98, 1975.

13. Hytten, FE and Baird, D: The development of the nipple in pregnancy, Lancet, 1201, 1958.

14. Otte, MJ: Correction inverted nipples-an aid to breast feeding, Am. J. Nurs. 75:454, 1975.

15. Hoffman, JB: Suggested treatment for inverted nipples, Am. J. Obstet. Gynecol. 66: 346, 1953.

16. Applebaum, RM: Breast feeding and care of the breasts, Chapter 32 in Davis, *Gynecology and Obstetrics,* Vol. 1. Hagerstown, Maryland: Harper & Row, Inc., 1974.

17. Blake, B et al: A Guide to Handling Breast-feeding Problems. Philadelphia: CEA of Greater Philadelphia, Spring 1977 edition.

18. Nipple Care. Franklin Park, Illinois: La Leche League International, 1978.

19. Confi-Dri milk cup for nursing mothers, CEA of Greater Philadelphia.

20. Egnell Co: Breast pump rental service. Cary, Illinois, Egnell, Inc., (Number 602).

21. Cotterman, J: Intensive preparation for inverted or retracting nipples, Keeping Abreast Journal I (4):330, 1976.

22. Brazelton, TB: Psychophysiologic reactions in the neonnate, J. Pediatr. 58:513, 1961.

23. Countryman, BA: How the maternity nurse can help the breastfeeding mother. Franklin Park, Illinois: La Leche League International, 1977.

24. Hellman, LM et al: *Williams Obstetrics,* New York: Appleton-Century Crofts, 1971, p. 993.

25. Rice, I: *Heartstart: A Practical Guide to Breastfeeding.* St. Paul: Ilene Rice, 2392 Nancy Place, St. Paul, Minn. 1977.

26. Marshall, BR et al: Sporadic puerperal mastitis, JAMA, 223, Sept. 29, 1975.

27. Niebyl, JR et al: Sporadic (nonepidemic) puerperal mastitis, J. Reprod. Med. 20 (2):97, 1978.

Chapter 9

The Learning Period

GENERAL DISCUSSION

The pediatrician or other health professional who cares for the infant has not traditionally been involved with caring for the infant's mother. Success at breastfeeding, however, requires supporting the mother, especially during the early weeks of lactation. Supporting the nursing couple requires a change in focus from the baby to the mother and her interaction with her infant. It also requires an understanding of the new mother's situation in the early weeks.

The term "the learning period" has been aptly used to describe the first six weeks of lactation, during which the new mother is learning to breastfeed (1). The learning period is of crucial importance. Early lactation failure, which is not uncommon, happens during this period and is the result of an inadequate understanding of breastfeeding, confusion about normal infant behaviors or lack of emotional support of the new mother by those around her. An understanding of the mind set of the new mother is helpful to anyone who wants to foster successful breastfeeding and thus will be described in this chapter.

Ideally the basic principles of breastfeeding have been taught to the new mother during her hospital stay. Or she may have learned the principles by reading a book on breastfeeding or by attending the meetings of a breastfeeding group. How a new mother has learned the simple breastfeeding basics is not important, but without this understanding, a woman breastfeeding for the first time faces an almost impossibly difficult learning period.

How a new mother perceives herself and her baby during these first weeks influences greatly her confidence, and that affects her ability to relax and to enjoy her baby. The ability to relax and enjoy a newborn also requires that she understand normal newborn behavior. Her baby's needs are total, immediate, and sometimes seem to be without end.

The relation of the nursing couple to the family and especially to the father also is a factor during this special time. A father often feels excluded in the early postpartum period as the new mother's attention is shifted from him to the care of the newborn. There may be feelings of jealousy because of the close relationship between the nursing mother and child. Added to the sexual readjustments that occur during pregnancy and in the postpartum period (see Chapter 11) the new father's adjustment (or maladjustment) to the nursing infant may have a significant effect on the mother's confidence and success at breastfeeding. His support of the new mother is important.

BEHAVIOR OF THE NURSING NEWBORN
DURING THE LEARNING PERIOD

The common pattern of breastfed infants sleeping for short periods and awakening to nurse frequently has been described as "continuous" feeding and correlates with the low protein content and easy digestibility of the breast milk. It has been suggested that there is a relationship between the protein content and the frequency of feeds among different groups of mammals. Human milk, with low protein, puts man among species that need to be "continuously" fed (2). (See Chapter 2) In many cultures mother and baby never are separated, the mother carrying her young infant with her everywhere and offering the breast as comfort whenever the infant wakens and stirs. This pattern is unfamiliar to Western women, whose culturally based expectation is for long naps between feedings (more easily accomplished with higher protein formula feeds).

In Western cultures the mother puts her baby to the breast primarily for the purpose of giving him milk. Thus the mother feels free to withhold the breast if she supposes that the baby has had enough or is not hungry. This is profoundly different from the normal pattern of most cultures, in which the breast is offered not primarily for the purpose of getting milk into him, but to keep him comfortable and happy. Although the milk is incidental, in the process of frequent nursings, the baby gets all the milk he needs (1).

Night Feedings

In Western cultures, newborns are expected to have one night-feeding, the "two o'clock feeding" and to give up this feeding sometime in the first weeks or months. Some babies sleep through the night as soon as they come home from the hospital; others spontaneously give up night-feedings as expected. The remaining, who continue to wake, may be perceived as atypical or even abnormal. This attitude appears to reflect a cultural bias since the expectation of sleeping through the night is not universal for all cultures.

Various theories—all unproven—have been postulated to explain night wakefulness. In evolutionary terms, modern Western man is still basically a hunter-gatherer. In hunter-gatherer societies, the woman is an essential member of the group in food collecting or preparing activities. During the day she cannot stop for long leisurely nursings, so the daytime nursings are relatively brief and interspersed with activities that must continue. At night, when the group is settled, the mother and baby are able to enjoy long and leisurely nursings. The neonate in the modern Western world, who is in evolutionary terms no different from the baby of the hunterer-gatherer, seems intrinsically to want to nurse as much (or even more) at night as in the daytime.

Another theory is that during pregnancy, the mother was active during the day and her body motions lulled the fetus to sleep; at night, when movement stops, the fetus awakens. Many women report that when they lie down to sleep there is increased movement of the fetus.

In a study of sleeping customs in 186 cultures, not one culture followed the pattern preferred by Westerners—that the mother and father sleep together in a room that is separate from the baby (3).

In our culture as in others, then, the pattern of at least one night feeding is common and it often continues beyond first weeks and months. Encouraging a new mother, especially a first time mother, to nap during the day is especially helpful during the early weeks. In any event, the young breastfed infant may awaken one or more times to nurse through the night and these feedings are clearly normal.

The baby who seems to have days and nights confused, who awakens at night more often than during the day, should be encouraged to nurse more frequently during the day. The mother needs to awaken the baby during the day as often as every 2-2½ hours to nurse and also can encourage him to stay awake by playing, talking, carrying or bathing him after nursing or between nursings.

Growth Spurts

Mothers often describe periods of increased nursing that last about 48 hours. The baby seems to be continually hungry, and awakens even more frequently than usual, wanting to nurse. These periods are sometimes called growth spurts and frequently occur at the following approximate ages: 10-14 days, 4-6 weeks, 3 months, and 6 months (when solids are easily introduced). Experienced nursing mothers are less aware of growth spurts, perhaps reflecting their lack of concern with the number of feeds per day. Offering formula supplements interferes with the normal process of increasing the suckling time and, thereby milk supply, and should be discouraged during these times.

It is important to explain to mothers the normalcy of these periods, ideally before they occur and in terms that the mother can readily understand: "If you were bottle feeding and your baby was not satisfied with four ounces you could put six ounces in the bottle. You can't just get your breasts to produce more milk with words. But nursing frequently for about 48 hours will stimulate your breasts to produce more milk."

The baby's first growth spurt, which usually takes place around 10 days postpartum, is of special importance. Other things that are happening at the same time compound the new mother's concerns about her milk supply. Breast engorgement, the edema (but not the milk) of early lactation, is disappearing. In addition, the baby is likely to be sleeping less than he did in the first days postpartum and also is likely to be beginning to have a fussy period. He is not yet smiling. The combination of a growth spurt, flatter breasts, and a fussing baby has led many new mothers to think that they have lost their milk. Offering a formula supplement in this setting is often the first step in early weaning.

The second growth spurt is likely to occur at about 4 to 6 weeks, another common time at which women give up breastfeeding. In this case also, there are other factors that are compounding the problem. The mother no longer considers herself "postpartum" and is very likely to overtire herself trying to resume many of her activities. Also the time period around 4 to 6 weeks is likely to be marked by extreme fussiness in the baby, especially in the late afternoon or evening. Again, each breastfeeding mother can be spared anxiety by being forewarned about the second growth spurt along with not getting overtired and that she may need to give more frequent nursings for 48 hours to increase the milk supply.

Other Aspects of Early Breastfeeding

The following list enumerates normal aspects of early breastfeeding, which, because they are unfamiliar, are likely to be perceived by the new mother as problems. Sometimes she brings them to the physician's attention. All that is required is to reassure the mother of their normalcy. Additional suggestions are given in parentheses.

. . . . . . Normal Behavior During Early Breastfeeding. . . . . . .

1.   Baby often wants to nurse ONLY 1 ½ hours or whatever after the last feeding.

2.   Mother describes having less milk at the late afternoon feeding.

3.   Baby has very frequent stools, as often as after every feeding.

4.   Baby has only infrequent stools, once a week; they are large but soft.

5.   Mother complains of pain in her nipples at the beginning of each feeding which is relieved when the milk lets down (see Chapter 8).

6.   Mother describes a pain in the breast at the beginning of feedings only. (She is feeling a "powerful let-down")

7.   Baby gasps or seems to choke as the milk lets down forcefully. (The baby will soon be well able to handle this early flow and the problem resolves spontaneously)

8.   Baby does not burp after feedings. (Some breastfed babies do and some do not need to burp after feedings; the mother can be advised to lay the baby down on his side after the feeding.)

9.   Baby takes the nipple into his mouth, then lets go. A full breast may be blocking his nose so he cannot breathe. (Mother should depress an area of breast away from baby's nose with her finger.)

10.   Baby cannot stay awake to nurse at the second breast. (Mother can break suction after 10 minutes, change diaper, etc. to rouse the baby and offer the second breast. She can try to divide whatever amount of time baby does nurse between both breasts.)

The following are also found with bottle fed babies; again, what is indicated is reassurance that this too is normal.

11.   Baby is fussy every evening.

12.   Baby spits up small amount of milk after feedings.

THE NEW MOTHER'S PERCEPTIONS
DURING THE LEARNING PERIOD

The new mother who has given birth to a healthy baby is proud, happy, relieved and widely congratulated. She is likely to be delighted with her beautiful baby.

Nevertheless the immediate postpartum period is often described by women as a blur. The mother of a two week old has been compared to a fatigued new intern. Even the experienced mother finds this period a difficult one.

In addition to physical recovery from childbirth, and readjustment of hormone levels, the mother is faced with the care of a totally dependent human being. She is in the state of becoming a mother ("matrescence"), which is at times a difficult process (see Chapter 1).

A key phrase that has helped many women through the learning period is that "Things will get better." The light at the end of the tunnel concept frequently is helpful when it is enunciated to the new mother by the physician, nurse or breastfeeding counselor. Understanding that the seemingly endless middle of the night feeds decrease in number with time, that sore nipples get better, that with each day the mother is learning to know her own infant's needs better can help a new mother to feel that her ceaseless efforts are worthwhile.

A sense of isolation may first occur when whatever help was available during the day (grandmother, husband) leaves. The new mother is suddenly left alone with the complete care of the newborn. She is stuck at home in what Brazelton has called an "almost impossible" situation for which she was in no way prepared (4).

Many mothers of first babies have a limited knowledge of mothering skills as well as of breastfeeding. In years of schooling, even in prepared childbirth classes, little or no information about mothering is given. Even the simplest techniques that are effective in soothing infants, such as swaddling, rocking, and suckling, are rarely discussed with young mothers of first babies, who must then discover them for themselves (2).

Although crying in infancy is a normal occurrence, the new mother's perception of the crying may lead to difficulties. Breastfeeding mothers are likely to attribute their babies' crying to hunger, while bottle feeding mothers attribute the crying to various other causes, such as gas, crabbiness, etc. In one study, many of the breastfeeding mothers gave up nursing because of a mistaken belief that crying denotes an inadequate milk supply (5).

The new mother who is trying conscientiously to find the cause of her baby's crying does not realize that it is sometimes impossible to determine the source of the distress. Nor does the new mother realize that "if something *stops* a baby crying (e.g., being given milk or the return of the mother) the lack of milk or mother may not have originally caused the crying. (2)" The fact that offering the breast soothes the crying baby does not necessarily prove that hunger was the original cause of the crying, especially since nursing provides the mother's attention, her warmth, the sound of her heartbeat, sucking satisfaction, and food.

Comforting the Crying Baby

When comfort for a crying or fussy baby is needed, solutions other than nursing most often are suggested in Western cultures. It is certainly helpful for the new mother and father to learn how to swaddle their baby, to hold him up to the shoulder, to rock him, to talk to him, to play with him. Babies have needs other than breastfeeding, which parents are learning during the early weeks. But giving a bottle of water or supplemental formula, offering a pacifier or pushing the carriage back and forth have an advantage that may explain why they are commonly recommended. They allow baby nurses, grandmothers, or fathers to participate more directly in care-giving activities, from which they are excluded with breastfeeding. It is not surprising that nursing is less commonly recommended as a soothing technique in Western cultures, although it is an easy and effective technique and ought not to be overlooked. Other soothing techniques (see Chapter 10) can be suggested to mothers who request information on what to do with the fussy baby.

Concerns about "spoiling" the baby are not uncommon and reflect in large part a lack of understanding of normal child development in infancy.

Styles of Breastfeeding

In addition to learning about mothering, which is a task for all mothers breast- or bottle feeding, the breastfeeding mother must also learn *how to* breastfeed. Unlike simpler cultures in which all women nurse in the same approximate style, Western culture in the twentieth century has evolved different styles of breastfeeding.

The following quotation describes the evolution of a style of breastfeeding that is so unfamiliar to many Westerners:

> When a woman breast feeds, she must give herself to the baby. She must let the baby set the pace, make the decisions, do the work. Many mothers cannot do this at first, especially if they have been handed (or have asked for) a fixed set of rules. But the normal girl eventually gets "lazy" and slips into the feminine role. She forgets to look at the clock, she doesn't worry about when or why he wants to eat. She actively gives the baby her milk and her love, whenever he seems to want it. She lets him move around, start and stop, nurse at his own rate, interrupt his meals, or, when she has leisure, prolong them. She learns to participate in feedings

without dominating or deciding anything, to be deeply interested but quite casual about the whole matter. This is the
natural result of successful breast feeding, no matter what
kind of personality the mother has. The woman who cannot
develop this completely casual approach with the first baby
often adopts it with her second; that is one reason why many
nursing mothers "have more milk" the second time around.
And even the most managing of women can often learn how
to breast feed in a natural, relaxed way from contact with
other mothers who are nursing successfully (1).

The mode described above has been called normal unrestricted or successful breastfeeding (6); in this style of total breastfeeding, the breast is
offered for comfort as well as for food according to the infant's needs.

An objection to this pattern of frequent unscheduled nursings is that
Western women have other responsibilities. "Demand" feeding is perceived
as too tiring for the busy modern woman, although most women in the first
six weeks postpartum, whether they are breast-or bottle feeding, are mainly
engaged in postpartum readjustment and in caring for the baby. In an attempt to spare the new mother from too much nursing, she may be told not
to nurse too often or to nurse only to allay hunger. Thus, a style of breastfeeding has evolved in which women withhold the breast for comfort and
offer it only for food. The admonition to "try to get him on a schedule"
or not to nurse any more often than every three hours, although counter-
productive to successful nursing is still widely made.

A common Western style of breastfeeding by rules (on when to feed, on
the mother's lifestyle, etc.) is sometimes called "modified breastfeeding,"
"token breastfeeding," "supplemented breastfeeding," "not being fanatical
about breastfeeding," and "modern breastfeeding." Regardless of the term
used, regulating early breastfeeding with rules or advising new mothers to
hold off nursing until a given time interval has passed makes life *more*
difficult for the mother. Substituting other care-giving activities (walking,
rocking, or giving a pacifier or water bottle), when one is faced with the
reality of the crying infant often is more tiring than just nursing. More serious problems with this style of nursing are that often the let-down reflex
may not be conditioned, and often women nurse too infrequently to maintain an adequate milk supply; early weaning is common (6).

There are many variations of styles of breastfeeding between the two
extremes described—unrestricted breastfeeding and modified breastfeeding.
The style that each mother adopts is usually based on what she learned
about child rearing as she grew up, what her family, friends, and people
in the medical profession, or members of a breastfeeding support group
are telling her now.

The Discouraged Mother

Occasionally one sees an overly conscientious new mother who may be nursing every 1½ - 2 hours, with feedings averaging 40 minutes in duration; she is likely to be feeling overwhelmed and exhausted. The mother who is becoming discouraged can be advised that while frequent nursings are appropriate, these need not continue more than 20 minutes. A pattern of "short frequent nursings" is better for the discouraged mother than a pattern of long infrequent nursings. This situation also is intensified by unnecessary nipple-washing and cream-applying routines, and overly elaborate hand-washing, and diaper-changing procedures. In some cases, the baby's weight gain also is poor. Gentle questioning about her let-down reflex may be in order, as such women often have difficulty relaxing.

The Mother Who is a Clock-Watcher

Women who have lived their whole lives according to fairly rigid scheduling find it difficult or impossible to forget the clock. Although the baby does not need a schedule, the mother clearly does. A mother who prefers a scheduled life-style may or may not be able to relax and forego clock-watching.

A woman who is insistent about getting her baby on a schedule can begin by writing down the baby's own pattern for a day or two. Is he wanting to nurse every 2 or 2½ or 3 hours? Does he have one long sleep time during the day or night? If the mother feels she must encourage her baby to nurse on some kind of schedule, she will be more successful if she picks one that is fairly close to the time interval her baby already has between feedings.

Mothers who want a schedule also find that devices such as bottles of water, pacifiers, or wind-up swings are useful. There are some women who breastfeed successfully on a schedule, although they are a minority.

SUPPORTING THE NEW MOTHER

The New Father as a Doula

If the woman is living with the father of the baby he can be extremely helpful in giving her encouragement and moral support. The new mother is in an emotionally dependent position and needs to be mothered. Even a young father who has little factual information about breastfeeding is likely to be pleased by the sight of his child happily nursing at the breast, and he often is the only person in the home to offer encouragement and to shield his wife from her own doubts and those of other people.

The new mother not only needs encouragement, she also needs help in specific areas.

...... The Father's Role During the Learning Period ......

1.   Adjusting to his own new role, and resolving his feelings about fatherhood, including feelings about breastfeeding

2.   Helping the mother to gain confidence about parenting and about breastfeeding

3.   Helping with other siblings, if there are any.

4.   Helping with food preparation.

5.   Helping to care for the household.

Although doulas have traditionally been female, a supportive husband is sometimes a more effective and loving doula for his wife than a female relative.

Although a strongly enthusiastic husband is ideal, in reality many fathers could be described as lukewarm supporters—but breastfeeding does continue. It is the negative or disapproving husband who makes successful breastfeeding nearly impossible. (A disagreement over breastfeeding may reflect a basic disagreement within a relationship).

Breastfeeding Support Groups

Attending the meetings of a support group or occasionally calling a friend who has breastfed successfully with questions or just to chat is especially helpful to a new mother. The opportunity to discuss her particular concerns with women of experience is useful. When talking with another mother who has nursed, the remark that the new mother may cherish most is simply "My baby did that too" or "I noticed that when my baby was that age."

Telephone Contact During the Learning Period

Making a telephone call to a new mother who is learning how to breastfeed is an effective way of preventing lactation failure. Telephone contact is particularly indicated when other suggested routes for conveying basic breastfeeding information are not practical (when little in-hospital teaching has taken place, or when the first well-baby check-up is not scheduled before 4 weeks).

The phone call is ideally made when the baby is 8-10 days old. It can be made by a nurse, a nurse practitioner (7), or a breastfeeding counselor. There are two main purposes of the call: [1] to help the new mother learn about breastfeeding, and [2] to detect potential problem areas early.

The idea of giving a mini-lesson on breastfeeding in a relatively brief telephone call may seem unfamiliar, but has been used very successfully by lay groups, especially by groups in which the breastfeeding counselor initiates a call to every new breastfeeding mother who has expressed interest in receiving help. The person who initiates the call usually begins by asking how the nursings are going. She can then give advice appropriate to the problems mentioned. She continues then to tell the new mother general things about early breastfeeding ("I would like to tell you about growth spurts").

The important "lessons" of the telephone call are similar to those that might have been conveyed through in-hospital teaching (see Chapter 6).

Checklist of Points to Remind Mothers About
. . . . .At 1-2 Weeks Postpartum . . . .

1. Milk production depends on sucking stimulation, including during periods of growth spurts. "The more you nurse, the more milk you will have."

2. The normal and easiest pattern is demand feeding, that the average number of feedings per 24 hours is 10. ("Clock-watching" is counter-productive and may interfere with the mother's relaxing.)

3. It is normal and advantageous for the new mother to offer the breast as comfort.

The second main purpose of the phone call is to detect early breastfeeding problems, and if appropriate, to recommend that the new mother bring her baby into the office for a check-up right away. In most cases all is well, and the new mother can be reassured and her questions answered. Occasionally the mother's remarks indicate a problem area which should be pursued.

. . . . . Warning Signs of Early Breastfeeding Problems . . . . . .

1. The baby is "so good," and rarely cries.

2. There are fewer than 7 nursings in a 24 hour period.

3. The mother has painfully sore nipples, a plugged duct, or some other breast problem.

4. The mother sounds extremely anxious.

Another system that is also very effective in guaranteeing that the nursing couple will receive breastfeeding help when it is most needed, early in the postpartum period involves scheduling the first check-up at approximately two weeks postpartum.

References

1.   Pryor, K: *Nursing Your Baby.* New York: Pocket Book Division of Simon and Schuster, 1973.

2.   Dunn, J: *Distress and Comfort.* Cambridge, MA: Harvard University Press, 1977.

3.   Barry, H, III and Paxson, LM: Infancy and Early Childhood: Cross Cultural Codes 2, Ethnology 10, 1971.

4.   Brazelton, JB, interview in Glickman, BM and Springer, BNB: *Who Cares for the Baby?* New York: Schocken Books, 1978.

5.   Bernal, JF: Crying during the first ten days and maternal responses, Dev. Med. Child. Neurology 14 362, 1972.

6.   Newton, N: *Maternal Emotions.* New York: Paul B. Hoeber, Inc., 1955.

7.   Selby, M: Fostering breastfeeding: a pediatric program, Keeping Abreast J. II (3):180, 1977.

Chapter 10

The Care of the Breastfed Baby

THE TWO-WEEK CHECK-UP

There are many advantages in making a first well-baby visit at two weeks of age. By then the mother and baby probably are beginning to feel more at ease and to be getting acquainted with each other. Most often the baby is gaining weight and doing well. Reassurance and praise can be given to the mother. Questions about routine baby care, as well as specifics about breast-feeding, are often formulated and can ideally be answered then. The baby's weight can be checked and compared with the hospital discharge weight. The ten-percent weight loss allowed by most sources in the first week of life may be a liberal allowance if babies are breastfed early and persistently.

At this visit the physician or nurse is able to pick up early nursing problems and, especially and most seriously, early signs of failure to thrive. Underfeeding can be suspected in infants who are making inadequate weight gain.

At the visit the physician or nurse needs to review frequency and length of feeds. If there is a question of adequacy of weight gain, nursing routines should be investigated further. Signs and symptoms of the let-down can be sought. It is sometimes useful to have an experienced observer watch a nursing. Is the baby properly placed at the breast? Is the nipple easily grasped? Is baby sucking vigorously? Is he content after a feeding, and is mother comfortable? Often an experienced female nurse may be useful here, as the mother may be uncomfortable nursing in front of a male physician, especially at this early stage of lactation. Care should be taken in discussing signs and symptoms of let-down to avoid overly concerning an already nervous or unsure mother.

The two-week check-up is an appropriate opportunity to explain and forewarn all mothers of growth spurts.

A truly underfed baby may be difficult to differentiate from a slow gainer at this point, and close follow-up is in order. Some breastfed babies gain
slowly, no matter how often or how long they are nursed. During the second
half of the first year and the beginning of the second year their weight seems
to catch up with height measurements. These children appear to be healthy
and well and represent a normal variation in infant growth patterns. The
differentiation of failure to thrive from slow weight gain may continue to be
difficult well into the early months of infancy.

If there are specific nursing problems—erratic let-down, a dissatisfied
infant—decreased milk supply should be suspected, and further intervention
is appropriate.

Low Weight Gain

When assessing a breastfed infant with a fairly low weight gain, it is appropriate to determine whether this is an infant who has a normal growth rate,
and who is being breastfed adequately (the normal slow gainer), or whether
the low weight gain is the result of a mother's inadequate milk supply (the
underfed infant). The following points can be checked in making an assess-
ment:

Differentiating Between a Slow Gaining Infant
. . . . and an Underfed Infant . . . .

Normal Slow Gainer	*Underfed Infant*
Baby appears to be alert and healthy	Infant appears either apathetic or cries for much of the day.
Good muscle tone	Infant may appear to be mildly dehydrated.
The skin obviously is smooth and healthy	
Many wet diapers (at least 6 per day), although the use of water bottles invalidates this observation.	Few wet diapers
Pale, unconcentrated urine	Strong urine
Stools very frequent—or if infre-quent, large, but soft	Stools infrequent, scanty

Infant nurses at least 8 times per day, in first month of life. Nursings generally are relaxed and continue for 15-20 minutes	Infant has fewer than 8 feedings per day, when the number is counted. Nursings often are brief.
The mother's let-down is functioning, she can describe some, if not all, signs of a functioning let-down (leaking, milk spurting, tingling, uterine contractions, thirst at onset of feeding, change in infant's swallowing pattern).	No signs of a functioning let-down when the mother is asked.
The pattern of weight gain is consistent, although low.	The baby may not gain weight, or the weight gain may be erratic (the infant may loose weight, gain a little, then loose).
The breast is being offered as comfort as well as nourishment.	The breast is not being offered as comfort; instead, a pacifier may be offered to satisfy sucking needs.

It is sometimes very time-consuming to determine the cause of poor weight gain and to recommend corrective measures. The reason that the two week check-up is an ideal time to identify problems is that, after the passage of time, problems often intensify: maternal frustration increases, and behaviors of the mother and baby are harder to change. Suggesting formula supplements is fast and easy advice and often will succeed in increasing weight gain. It is, however, most often not the best solution. The mother is likely to be left with feelings of guilt and/or inadequacy, especially if she truly wanted to breastfeed. In the following section, failure to thrive as related to breastfeeding is discussed with specific suggestions for management.

FAILURE TO THRIVE IN THE BREASTFEEDING INFANT
Failure to thrive at the breast is most often the result of insufficient milk supply. It is a curable problem for an otherwise well mother and baby, but must of course be differentiated from the many other causes for failure to thrive in infancy. The alert, skinny baby who has no signs of systemic disease at the two week visit can be assumed most often to be receiving too

little milk. Most often the problem is with the mother and not with the infant.

If one is to help the mother it is necessary to determine the factors causing an inadequate milk supply. Most often there is a problem with nursing skills, but, factors involving the mother's or infant's health need to be considered also.

Most Common Cause: Poor Nursing Skills

Failure to thrive at the breast usually is the result of poor nursing skills or poor let-down reflex. In many cases, the mother has been following a fixed and/or a limited schedule. She may be nursing as infrequently as 5 or 6 times in a 24 hour period, instead of the normal 8 to 12 feeds. (On the average, 10 feedings per 24 hours are expected in the first month.)

A good procedure is to instruct the mother whose baby has gained little or no weight to write down the frequency and duration of each feeding in the previous 24 hours. A mother's statement that she nurses "all the time" may actually reflect a limited schedule. The mother who is a clock-watcher, who holds the nursings to a set schedule, should be advised to nurse on demand.

Since a functioning let-down also is essential to successful lactation, and therefore to proper weight gain, the signs of a functioning let-down should be sought through gentle questioning so as not to alarm her. She may be asked about a change in infant's swallowing pattern, leaking during nursing, spurting milk, or nipple pain at onset of nursing. Most mothers will describe one or more of these signs of a functioning let-down (see also Chapter 8). Many women do not have all the signs, but a woman who reports no signs can be further asked if the nighttime feedings go more smoothly than the daytime feedings (nervous mothers relax better when they are alone and sleepy), and if the baby acts content after a nursing (If the baby is content after a feeding, the let-down is probably functioning; the baby is getting at least some milk).

Although failure to nurse frequently enough and/or failure to condition the let-down reflex to the nursing baby are the most common causes for poor weight gain in Western society, other factors must not be overlooked.

Failure to Thrive: Factors Involving the Mother

1. *Malnutrition.* If the mother is malnourished, she will continue to lactate, but her total milk yield will be diminished slightly. The extremely malnourished mother, however, often is unable to supply sufficient calories for her infant. It has been shown that improving maternal diet in this situation will result in increased milk supply and improved growth of the baby (1). Mal-

nourished mothers may need to add solids to the infant's diet earlier. This is a rare problem in the Western world, but not uncommon in poorer countries (2).

2. *Maternal Illness.* The woman with undiagnosed medical disease, such as an endocrinopathy, may produce insufficient milk. Optimal lactation requires normal levels of cortisone, thyroid hormone, parathyroid hormone and insulin. When kept in normal hormonal balance by proper medical treatment, however, the woman with an endocrinopathy can be expected to lactate normally and can be encouraged to breastfeed. Maternal illness should be looked for when nursing techniques appear to be optimal but the infant is failing to thrive and there are no signs of systemic disease within the infant.

3. *Vitamin Deficiency.* Any maternal vitamin deficiency eventually will cause a deficiency in the mother's milk. Initially, concentrations of vitamins and minerals remain constant in milk, but as maternal stores are depleted, milk becomes deficient. The most common maternal vitamin and mineral deficiencies are in iron and vitamin C. In a strict vegetarian—a vegan who, in addition to shunning meat and fish, does not eat milk, eggs, or cheese—vitamin B_{12} deficiency is likely to occur, given sufficient time. This may be associated with retarded growth and development in the breastfed infant. Vitamin and mineral supplements should be prescribed and dietary needs discussed with women with deficient diets (see Chapter 11).

4. *Medications.* The effect of maternal medications on milk supply also should be considered. Alcohol and nicotine are the most common offenders. If the mother is on any medication, even those generally felt to be safe for nursing babies, the possibility of a detrimental effect on the baby should be considered. Specifically, it may be appropriate to ask about use of marijuana, opiates and other illicit drugs.

Heavy smoking may lead to a decrease in milk production in some women. Nicotine has been detected in the milk of smoking mothers, and decreased milk production has been reported in mothers who smoke more than 20 to 30 cigarettes per day (3). Vomiting, abdominal cramping, and diarrhea may occur in the infant of the mother who smokes heavily (4).

5. *Improper Use of Devices.* The mother may have been using a breast or nipple shield throughout the feedings. (Mothers who do this rarely volunteer this information spontaneously.) If so, the shield should be eliminated (see Chapter 14).

The mother may be using a pacifier to comfort the infant after relatively brief feedings and therefore the total time spent in nursing is too short. In such cases, the pacifier should be eliminated.

Failure to Thrive: Factors Involving the Infant

As with bottle-fed infants, causes within the infant should always be considered. The differential diagnosis of true failure to thrive is all of pediatrics, and psychological factors must also be considered.

Common causes within the baby which may be picked up by history and physical examination at or before the two week check-up include congenital heart disease (murmur, cyanosis, signs of congestive failure); renal disease (abdominal mass, poor urinary stream); congenital infections (rash, hepatosplenomegaly, small head circumference); neurological disease (poor muscle tone, baby seems too sleepy, baby has a poor suck and/or swallow). Other rarer causes, such as metabolic and endocrine abnormalities, require further tests and there may be other signs and symptoms (vomiting, dehydration). The child who is obviously ill, or for whom the physician has great concern, may need to be hospitalized.

Increasing an Inadequate Milk Supply

The woman who wants to nurse her infant can be helped to improve what appears to be even a very inadequate milk supply. Keeping in touch with the mother to answer questions and to give reassurance must be arranged. Lay support groups are very valuable in this situation and should be encouraged, if the mother is agreeable, and one is available.

The infant who is failing to thrive should be seen again the following week for a weight check. A weight gain of 5 to 7 oz is acceptable, but close follow-up continues to be indicated until there is clear indication that the baby is truly thriving.

The woman must understand that the way to increase the milk supply is to increase nursing frequency and duration. Many women do not know that the average number of feedings in the first month is 10 per day, with both breasts offered at each feeding.

Each mother should also understand that neither good nutrition, nor a large intake of liquids, nor "Brewer's yeast," nor lots of rest guarantees an adequate milk supply. Without adequate stimulation of the breasts through nursing, such remedies are inadequate. Suggesting that the mother and baby get into bed together and stay there for several days is perhaps the best way to ensure more frequent nursing. The mother can be advised to get up only to go to the bathroom. She should try to pamper herself, watch TV (if she likes to), read, eat, drink, relax, *and nurse.* Helping her to arrange for house hold help may be vital; enlisting a husband or friend to help care for other children may be possible.

If the mother is unable or unwilling to get into bed with the baby, she should still be encouraged to make increased nursing the highest priority in her life, at least for a period of two days.

Supplements should be avoided except when there is real concern about adequate hydration. When the infant's condition requires hospitalization, the physician may consider hospitalization of both mother and child together. During this hospitalization, the mother can be encouraged to nurse frequently and she can be well cared for. Chloropromazine and oxytocin have been used in this setting (2) but are not necessary. Any supplements used should be given only after nursing and less frequently than nursing. As the milk supply increases, supplements should be eliminated one at a time. Using a Lact-Aid to supply supplements avoids the use of bottles and has been used successfully in this setting (5).

Women who reject suggestions that are made to them about changing their routines in order to increase the milk supply may not really be convinced that they want to breastfeed. Some of these women may prefer to bottle feed.

In other cases, the mother comes to understand the reasons behind her low milk supply but prefers not to change her routines. A woman whose life style involves much time away from home and her baby may come to the realization that breastfeeding is not for her. She would prefer to bottle feed.

Failure to thrive due to an inadequate milk supply can be largely prevented by instructing each new nursing mother about breastfeeding during her hospital stay. Women who have a basic understanding of breastfeeding, who nurse their infants on demand, and who are enjoying the experience, rarely have infants who fail to thrive. A well-motivated woman who really wants to nurse, who is well, and whose baby is normal, can be counted on to succeed if she is given adequate help, encouragement and consistent correct advice.

Obviously not all mothers do succeed. Often, after several weeks of effort by physician, nurse and/or lay counselor, regular supplements have to be added, and the mother shows relief. She really didn't want to nurse, but she felt she must try. In the 20th century Western World, such feelings are real, not uncommon, and not easily changed. She should be reassured that very adequate formulas are available and she should be helped to feel comfortable with the decision to formula-feed.

TYPES OF BABIES

It sometimes is useful to think of babies as falling into different categories, although a particular infant may not fit exactly into any. Mothers may raise questions about their infants' behavior and feeding patterns. The following section gives descriptions of types of babies and breastfeeding advice by type.

The Fat Baby

The truly obese infant whose weight is several standards of deviation above his length occasionally is being fully breastfed. At times the degree of obesity is sufficient to make intervention appropriate. This is an unusual occurence prior to the third or fourth month.

. . . . .Suggestions to Slow a Rapid Weight Gain . . . .

1.   Advise the mother to discontinue any supplemental solids.

2.   The mother can nurse on one breast instead of two at each feeding.

3.   She can try to keep feedings to not more often than every 2½-3 hours. Suggest that she use soothing and comforting techniques to comfort the baby between feeds.

4.   The mother can offer water between or after feedings.

The Colicky Baby

A truly colicky baby cries and appears to be in pain much of the time when he is awake. He often seems to have severe gas pains. He may draw his legs up, arch his back, and cry relentlessly. The cause of colic is not understood. Immaturity of the nervous and/or digestive systems is a widely accepted theory, because babies outgrow colic by about three months.

The mother is likely to feel inadequate and guilty and conscience striken. Recent emphasis on "good" mothering or "appropriate" mothering tends to cause feelings of blame and guilt for mothers whose babies cry a lot.

The mother of a colickly breastfed baby can be reassured that breast milk is the best and most easily digested infant food. Weaning to formula will not alleviate and may aggravate the problem.

Reassurance that the mother's feelings are normal and that the colic will pass with time is appropriate.

The baby who has fussy periods, most often in the evening, that may last as long as several hours is a normal baby. New mothers need reassurance that such fussy periods are common and normal. They do not represent inadequate mothering or inadequate milk supply.

Some babies are cranky (not actually colicky) intermittently all day. They rarely are underweight because of the response of mothers to offer the breast (or bottle) more frequently.

Somet-mes a mother can relate episodes of fussiness to her having eaten large amounts of a particular food (e.g., chocolate, acidic foods). If so, avoidance or moderation is appropriate. One or more suggestions from the following list can be made to the mother of a fussy baby.

. . . . .Soothing Techniques for a Fussy Baby . . . .

1. Trying to nurse in a quiet atmosphere.

2. Trying shorter, more frequent feeds, as often as every 1½ hours, using one breast per feeding. This avoids overfeeding, but allows frequent periods of comfort.

3. Holding the baby up to the shoulder during a walk so that the baby can look around.

4. Rubbing the baby's back, changing his diaper.

5. Swaddling the baby in a soft blanket.

6. Cuddling, stroking, holding, walking the baby.

7. Singing to the baby.

8. Laying the baby across mother or father's moving knees (This may be helpful during a meal).

9. Giving the baby an air bath.

10. Mother and baby taking a bath together.

11. Mother and baby sleeping or napping together, perhaps with baby lying across mother's chest.

12. Allowing the baby to cry himself to sleep—for a short period of time.

13. Using some pieces of equipment that are useful in soothing babies:
     (a) The rocking chair soothes the mother and baby together.
     (b) A car ride.

(c) A pacifier which soothes a baby who needs to suck but who doesn't need any more milk.

(d) A cloth baby carrier which is very useful during the typical fussy time of day, especially if the mother is trying to fix dinner. The mother carries her baby slung against her chest.

(e) Using music or the noise of a vacuum cleaner to soothe. Some mothers have made a tape recording of that noise. This is an idea similar to the records of the sound of the mother's heartbeat that are sold.

(f) A baby swing, a device some mothers like.

The Placid Baby

This baby is "so good." The "so good" baby often makes poor weight gain. He sleeps or lies quietly in the crib much of the day and night. The demand on the mother for nursing may be as infrequent as 4-6 times in 24 hours.

Often the mother believes that all is well until the first weight check. Rarely are there identifiable underlying causes, such as maternal or infant depressant medications, or neurological problems with the baby (e.g. Down's Syndrome). Most often no underlying causes are found. Advice concerning stimulating techniques may be appropriate.

. . . . . . .Techniques for Stimulating the Placid Baby . . . .

1.   Use of soothing techniques, such as swings or pacifiers, which interfere with the baby nursing effectively, should be avoided.

2.   Suggest that the mother increase body contact and skin contact and avoid leaving the baby alone in his crib when he is awake.

3.   Advise the mother to nurse frequently, at least every 2½ hours during daytime.

4.   Use jack-knifing (see Chapter 7).

5.   If the infant seems to fall asleep fairly soon after being put to the breast, suggest that the mother stroke him under the chin as he nurses. The stroking motion should be directed toward the mouth and be gentle but firm.

6.   Suggest that the mother change the baby's diaper after the first breast to rouse him enough to nurse on the second breast.

7. Suggest that the mother put a little cool water on the baby or that she undress him or loosen the blankets around him.

8. Suggest that the mother give the baby a bath before nursing.

The Easy Baby

The easy baby is different from the placid baby in that he is awake and alert, yet happy for much of the time. He nurses strongly and makes good weight gains. He does not have trouble staying awake at the breast. The easy baby nurses fairly frequently and has no difficulty in digesting breast milk, regardless of the mother's diet. He may not have any fussy period in the day and always is good natured.

The baby is a delight to his family. The mother needs reassurance that he is doing well and, like all mothers, can be reminded of the importance of her time spent with him between feedings. All babies need stimulation and this fellow may not demand it.

The Hospitalized Baby

The infant or toddler who requires hospitalization and who is nursing—like any hospitalized child, has special needs. Allowing and encouraging the nursing mother to stay with the child is appropriate. The child who is able to take fluids can be given no more nutritious food than his mother's milk, and in no more comforting manner than at his mother's breast.

Mothers have used their ingenuity to nurse babies who were in traction or restrained in the bed. Mothers whose babies were in oxygen tents have lain in the tents next to their babies for general comfort and in order to nurse.

References

1. Sosa, R et al: Feed the nursing mother, thereby the infant, J. Pediatr. 88:668, 1976.

2. Jelliffe, DB and Jelliffe, EFP: *Human Milk in the Modern World.* Oxford: Oxford University Press , 1978.

3. Hervada, A et al: Drugs in breast milk, Perinatal Care 2:19, 1978.

4. Vorherr, H: Drug excretion in breast milk, Postgraduate Medicine 56:97, 1974.

5. Weichert, CE: Lactational reflex recovery in breastfeeding failure, Pediatrics 63:799, 1979.

Chapter 11

Caring for the Lactating Woman

GENERAL DISCUSSION

After the birth of a child, the primary focus of care in Western culture most often shifts from the woman toward the baby. In fact, in some recent discussions of breastfeeding, concern for the mother and baby seems to have swung rather far toward the baby (1); the majority of new reports on breastfeeding seem to emphasize the advantages of breast milk for the infant and are in the pediatric and not the obstetrical literature. Yet for breastfeeding to be successful—for babies to actually experience the advantages of breast milk and for mothers to know the pleasures of breastfeeding—the new mother must be supported. (It also is of note that those who have been effective in nurturing successful breastfeeding for the greatest numbers of women—traditional doulas and lay groups—have focused their attention primarily on the mother and only indirectly on the baby.)

Often different physicians care for the mother and her breastfed child, and the mother may be unsure of which doctor's office to call with a breastfeeding problem, especially in the early weeks.

There are special concerns specific to the lactating woman which may begin with the initiation of lactation but continue well beyond the neonatal period. This chapter discusses caring for the breastfeeding woman as an individual distinct from the baby.

Related concerns for the health professionals who provide care for the woman are found in Chapter 8 (Breast Problems) and Chapter 3 (The Pharmacology of Drugs in Breast Milk).

MATERNAL NUTRITION DURING LACTATION

Present recommendations for the diet during lactation of well-nourished women are for an additional 500 Cal/day, which should include 20 g of protein and 500 mg of calcium. The caloric estimate assumes that an extra 3-4 kg of body weight is present postpartum that will be lost during the first 3-4 months of lactation (2). (See Table 11-1.) As milk supply increases, by 4-6 months caloric needs may increase.

This gives an idea of extra nutritional needs but is only an approximation. The teenager who is lactating may have greater caloric needs than a mature woman because of her own continuing growth.

The woman who neglects her diet or who attempts to lose weight quickly, especially in early lactation, is likely to notice increased fatigue and decreased stamina. A well-balanced diet is more important to the mother's well-being than to her milk supply, which will not be greatly affected.

The chronically malnourished woman has special needs and is unlikely to be receiving the ideal dietary allowances of Table 11-1. Decreased milk yields are likely, and breastfed infants under these circumstances will need supplemental foods before the 4-6 months recommended for the infants of well-nourished women. Vitamin deficiencies also are more likely to occur with malnutrition. The true vegan (no animal protein of any kind) is at risk for B_{12} deficiency herself along with her breastfed infant (3). There is, however, little change in protein and lactose concentration in the milk, regardless of the woman's nutritional status (see Chapter 2).

The woman eating a well-balanced diet does not need vitamin or mineral supplements, but if there is reason for concern about dietary adequacy of vitamins and minerals, these can be prescribed. Iron supplements are indicated if mother is deficient and are prescribed routinely in early lactation by many. Most important is the intake of enough calories. If a balanced diet is followed, eating to appetite generally results in adequate calorie intake, and a slow return to pre-pregnancy weight probably will occur. In Western culture where food is plentiful and overeating common, the effect of lactation on weight is variable; some women lose weight beyond that of pre-pregnancy while others have difficulty getting back to pre-pregnancy weight.

Moderation in alcohol intake is appropriate. Advice concerning an occasional glass of sherry or beer in late afternoon (which may help mother face the early evening fussy period) must be given carefully. Excessive amounts of alcohol are ill-advised and have been reported to cause a "pseudo-Cushing" syndrome, with excessive weight gain and poor growth in the infant (4).

Specific foods are sometimes assumed to cause increased fussiness in the nursing baby, especially foods such as garlic and onions whose volatile oils flavor the milk. The smell of onion or garlic can sometimes be detected on the nursing baby's breath, or when he burps after nursing, often the baby being perfectly happy. But if a baby acts fussy and his breath smells like

Table 11-1
Recommended Daily Dietary Allowances for Lactation
for Women Ages 23-50*

Body size	
Weight (kg)	58
(lb)	128
Height (cm)	162
(in)	65
Nutrients	
Energy (kcal)	2500
Protein (gm)	66
Vitamin A (retinol equivalants)	1200
(IU)	6000
Vitamin D (IU)	400
Vitamin E activity (IU)	15
Ascorbic Acid (mg)	80
Folic Acid (μg)	600
Niacin (mg**)	18
Riboflavin (mg)	1.7
Thiamine (mg)	1.3
Vitamin B_6 (mg)	2.5
Vitamin B_{12} (μg)	4.0
Calcium (mg)	1200
Phosphorus (mg)	1200
Iodine (μg)	150
Iron (mg)	18
Magnesium (mg)	450
Zinc (mg)	25

*Modified from Food and Nutrition Board. National Research Council, National Academy of Sciences: Recommended Dietary Allowances, ed. 8, Washington, D.C., 1974, Government Printing Office.

**Although allowances are expressed as niacin, it is recognized that on the average, 1 mg of niacin is derived from each 60 mg of dietary tryptophan.

onion, the assumption is made that the baby is reacting to the onion-flavored milk. This is not necessarily valid. If the baby is bothered *consistently* after the mother eats one particular food, there is more reason to blame the food.

Other foods such as chocolate are sometimes consistently associated with increased fussiness in the baby and can be avoided or taken only in moderation.

Sometimes the intake of caffeine as from great quantities of iced tea or coffee is associated with increased wakefulness in both mother and baby.

It is popularly believed, although not investigated, that many food substances that are ingested in large quantities by the mother may bother the baby through her milk. Foods that have been suspected are cows' milk, eggs, wheat—and any food for which there is a family history of allergy. No evidence exists to prove or disprove this possibility.

. . . . . .Suggested Dietary Guidelines during Lactation. . . . . .

1. Increased fluids: drink to thirst.

2. Protein: 3 or 4 servings/day of meat, fish, cheese, eggs, cottage cheese, peanut butter, or combinations of foods with incomplete proteins, such as beans and corn.

3. Calcium: cows' milk is a good source but other sources include cheese, dairy products, sardines, salmon, shrimp, kale, and calcium supplements.

4. Carbohydrates such as from whole grains: 2-4 servings/ day.

5. Fresh fruits and vegetables: 4-6 servings/day.

American women on limited incomes who wish to nurse their babies should be told of the help they can receive from community or government agencies. The Women, Infants and Children (WIC) program of the U.S. Department of Agriculture, provides nutritional guidance and food supplements for lactating women.

Diet at Weaning
Women sometimes gain weight after and during weaning. The caloric needs of lactation are greater so that at weaning well-nourished women need to cut back on their caloric intake to avoid excessive weight gain.

Contaminants in Human Milk
The possible danger to nursing babies from contaminants in the mothers' milk is a concern to some pregnant and lactating women (see Chapters 3 and 5). When there is a well-documented maternal exposure to a specific contaminant, as from certain polychlorinated biphenyls, (PCB's), contaminated game fish or other known sources, maternal blood levels could be measured (5).

Women who have become alarmed by television and newspaper stories but are not aware of any specific exposure sometimes ask if they should have their milk tested. No knowledgeable individuals or agencies have recommended the widespread testing of human milk.

An accurate testing of a mother's milk must be based on more than one sample. The milk should be pumped and collected from several sessions and must include the fatty hind milk. (Hand expressing a little of the fore milk would not be adequate for accurate testing of a fat soluble substance). There are few laboratories which are prepared to do this type of testing and there are no guidelines to interpret even accurate data.

A two-year study to compare environmental contaminants ingested by breastfed and bottle-fed babies now is being conducted by the National Institute of Environmental Health Science (7). Some women may need to be reassured that the possible dangers are generally considered to be out-weighed by the proven advantages of breast milk.

. . . . Suggestions for Reducing Intake of Contaminants. . . . .

1.   Avoid the use of all pesticides. Use a fly swatter or, in the garden, biological methods. Home grown fruits and vege-tables can be raised without pesticides or one can buy only those which have not been sprayed.

2.   Avoid going to places where such chemicals are used, such as orchards sprayed with pesticides. Avoid working at an occupation in which there is exposure to dangerous chem-icals.

3.   Avoid any food which would be likely to have chemical contamination, especially predatory fresh-water fish from contaminated waters.

4.   Avoid being on reducing diets during lactation, espe-cially one that might cause a fairly rapid weight loss. Con-taminants are stored in body fat and can be released in milk fat when fat is shed.

5.   Wash all fruits and vegetables thoroughly before eating.

6.   Since chemicals in meat are concentrated in the fat, cut off and discard all fat from meat.

7.   Limit the consumption of animal fats, especially red meats and butter. (These foods are at the top of the food chain and contain higher levels of contaminants.) A woman who is interested in a serious change in her dietary habits can be referred to Lappé: *Diet For A Small Planet* (6).

8. Eliminate or cut down on smoking; tobacco plants are sprayed with pesticides.

INFERTILITY AND SEXUALITY

Infertility

Breastfeeding can be shown epidemiologically to prolong the period of infertility postpartum and is perhaps the most effective form of birth control on a world-wide basis (8). The duration of lactational infertility varies considerably among various populations of women. Lactational amenorrhea, the period during which menstruation is suppressed, is easier to note than the duration of lactational anovulation (and infertility) during which ovulation (and therefore fertility) is suppressed. Among Western women, the average duration of lactational amenorrhea has been reported to vary between a relatively brief period of 88 days (9) to as long as 14.6 months among women who meet all of the baby's needs for food and comfort with long nursings day and night (10).

The median duration of lactational amenorrhea also varies among non-Western women; it was found to be more than two years on the average in rural areas of Zaire, Indonesia, and Bangladesh, and about 12 months in India, Taiwan, and South Korea (11). Various factors have been suggested to be responsible for this wide range, including the following:

Some Causes of Lactational Infertility
. . . . and Amenorrhea. . . . .

1. Hormonal effects of suckling

2. Style of breastfeeding

3. Maternal nutrition

4. Supplemental feedings

5. Traditional taboos on intercourse during lactation

6. Urbanization

7. Maternal age

Hormonal Effects of Lactation
During the immediate period postpartum, there is a period of infertility in both breast- and bottle feeding women. This is believed to be caused by

[1] an unresponsiveness of the ovaries to the pituitary gonadotropins which are required to trigger ovulation (luteinizing hormone or LH and follicular-stimulating hormone or FSH) but which are secreted and/or [2] to decreased secretion during this period of these pituitary gonadotropins (9). The exact mechanism is unknown. This effect lasts about 6 weeks in non-lactating women. During lactation, there appears to be further suppression of ovulation related to prolactin secretion. An inverse relation between prolactin secretion and gonadotropin levels can be demonstrated (9). That is, secretion of prolactin appears to depress secretion of FSH and LH. Women who are fully breastfeeding without use of supplemental feeds and who nurse frequently and through the night tend to have and, to maintain, slightly higher baseline levels of prolactin than women who are partially breastfeeding (12). The surges of prolactin that occur during nursing (and to a lesser extent during pumping or hand expression of milk) are in most studies present only during the first months of nursing, but probably continue longer when nursing is total nutrition and is on a demand schedule day and night.

The higher levels of prolactin may, in addition to suppression of secretion of gonadotropins, have a direct effect on the ovary. There may be suppression of luteal function as a direct effect of prolactin, with resulting decreased secretion of estrogen by the ovaries (9).

Much of the confusion about the duration of lactational amenorrhea is related to the lack of a clear definition of breastfeeding. "Full breastfeeding" means that no complementary foods of any kind are given to the infant and frequent nursings are given day and night. In some cultures, it is common for the mother and baby to sleep together, and for the baby to nurse many times during the night, even while the mother is sleeping. In this setting, baseline prolactin levels may be higher and persist longer. When a mother and baby sleep separately, and the mother is not exposed to suckling during the night, the plasma concentration of prolactin does not rise (as it does episodically during each nursing) which may allow a breakthrough surge of gonadotropins followed by ovulation (9).

The intensity of suckling also affects prolactin secretion. The mother nursing twins simultaneously has a rise in prolactin double that observed when one baby nurses (9).

Malnutrition, which by itself may cause decreased fertility (e.g., loss of menses during anorexia nervosa) may also have an effect on the style of breastfeeding. The infant who is nursing from a malnourished mother obtains a smaller amount of milk. Therefore suckling will be more intense, with longer bouts of suckling at shorter intervals. The infant must use more intense suckling and more bouts of suckling in order to maintain appropriate nutrition; this increased suckling may increase the contraceptive effect of nursing through a higher prolactin secretion (8).

In those cultures or sub-cultures where breastfeeding is total and lengthy feeds are frequent throughout the day and night, menstruation and ovulation appear the most delayed even among well-nourished women. Such is the case with women who are affiliated with a breastfeeding support group such as La Leche League (13). Many reports of an anecdotal type from women affiliated with another large breastfeeding support group suggest that many women begin to menstruate only after solid foods are introduced, and reports of lactational amenorrhea lasting for 9-18 months are not uncommon (14).

In addition to these hormonal effects related to style of breastfeeding and to maternal nutrition, the effects of cultural taboos on intercourse during lactation also are a factor. A period of abstinence from sexual intercourse is not uncommon in many non-Western cultures and may vary from several months through the duration of nursing. The period of lactational amenorrhea appears to correlate with duration of breastfeeding (15,16).

The resumption and then subsequent suppression of the menstrual cycle in a lactating woman is another phenomenon that is not clearly understood. It has generally been assumed that once menstruation has resumed postpartum in a lactating woman, the cycles will continue normally, although it is recognized that various factors (emotional, nutritional) can interrupt the menstrual cycle in any woman, lactating or not. However a marked change in nursing pattern also appears to be capable of interrupting the cycle temporarily. One woman, whose menstrual periods had resumed at 3½ to 4 weeks after the birth of each of her 6 children, changed her usual nursing pattern from brief nursings to long nursings after the sixth pregnancy. Her menstrual periods then stopped at 4 months postpartum and lactational amenorrhea continued for an additional 4 months (10). Although this one report in the literature is in no way conclusive, and other factors also may have been present, many other women have made (unpublished) reports that a drastic change in the nursing pattern temporarily interrupted their menstrual cycle. Women who have typically resumed menstruation when nursings were decreased in frequency and duration (during the 4-6 month period when babies are easily distracted, or after solid foods were introduced) occasionally change their nursing pattern to one of long, frequent nursings in the later part of the first year (because of illness, teething, separation anxiety, nighttime wakefulness) and they sometimes find that their menstrual cycle is delayed. Further study is clearly needed, with consideration of all possible contributing factors.

An interesting, although unstudied, observation of the effect of suckling and lactation on menstruation can be seen in the experiences of adoptive mothers. Women who attempt to induce lactation often report that induced lactation appears to affect the menstrual cycle. "Menses in most women occurred at longer intervals, and flow was diminished and of shorter duration than prior to lactation. A few mothers noted no change in normal menstrual patterns." (17)

Some, although not all, women who resume menstruation while they are still nursing observe that their babies do not want to nurse during the menstrual periods. The fussiness noted in some babies has led to the opinion that the babies simply are reacting to mood changes in the mother, although a decrease in the amount of milk produced is a possible explanation. Whether the milk actually tastes different—as many women firmly believe—has not been determined.

Contraception During Lactation

The duration of lactational infertility in an individual woman is not possible to predict. The first ovulation sometimes precedes the first menstrual period, making pregnancy possible before the return of menses. Some women are unaware of this possibility. Lactation is best viewed as postponing, rather than as preventing, pregnancy. This is not an adequate or acceptable form of contraception for the majority of Western women, and a surer form of contraception is necessary. With the possible exception of some oral contraceptives, any of the forms of contraception are appropriately prescribed when contraception is requested.

Lactating women whose religious or personal beliefs prohibit any form of artificial birth control, however, often find the period of lactational amenorrhea a difficult one if they do not want to conceive again. Particularly in need of help are those women who have been accustomed to using the rhythm or calendar method to keep track of fertile periods during which sexual abstinence must be practiced. Many women have reported that, although they enjoyed breastfeeding and the baby was thriving, they weaned to a bottle between two and four months in order that they might have regular menstrual periods as a guide to preventing pregnancy. Other women have reported that they have observed a practice of nearly total abstinence during the time when they knew that a return to fertility was possible; not infrequently, this is a period of several months. Clearly, these women have not been helped with common and traditional methods.

Some couples who are opposed to any form of artificial birth control may wish to follow the plan described in *Breast Feeding and Natural Child Spacing* (10), by which very frequent and lengthy feedings day and night postpone the return of fertility. Other couples, however, especially those who already have several children, or who want very much to prevent pregnancy (not postpone it) will not find such a plan satisfactory.

The Ovulation Method (also called the Billings Method) (18) can be considered for women who are opposed to artificial birth control and who want to prevent pregnancy during the period of lactational amenorrhea. Women are thereby taught to recognize different types of cervical mucus. The appearance of "fertile" mucus (clear, slippery, stretchy and like the raw white of an egg) signals that ovulation will be occurring relatively soon, and sexual intercourse must be avoided for the next few days. Dr. Billings recommends that the lactating woman begin checking at three weeks postpartum, although she may have to be watching for many weeks or months prior to the return of fertility.

In The Sympto-Thermic Method (19) the woman notes any variation in her temperature, in addition to checking the cervical mucus, as possible clues to returning fertility.

These methods require a great deal of time, patience and cooperation— and may be less reliable than conventional methods.

Sexuality

The effect of early lactation on sexuality is an area of clinical importance. One point of conjecture and some disagreement is the question of how lactation affects the woman's libido. Most often referred to is the Masters and Johnson report on postpartum women in *Human Sexual Response* (20). Masters and Johnson found in studying three postpartum nursing women and interviewing 24 postpartum nursing women, that breastfeeding women described an interest in a more rapid return to coition than did non-nursing women. While Masters and Johnson's finding often has been quoted, their associated remarks and findings on this subject have been largely ignored. When quoted in isolation from other salient points, the statement that the nursing women were more interested in resuming intercourse appears to have a somewhat different meaning than when the comment is studied in context. The higher level of sexual interest is no more significant than other findings, that a return to intercourse by nursing mothers was sometimes prompted by guilt over being sexually stimulated by the nursing infant, and that many women were motivated at least partially by concern for releasing their husbands' levels of sexual tensions.

An interview was held by Masters and Johnson in the third month postpartum with 110 postpartum women, 24 of whom were nursing.

> Ten women from the previously nulliparous group and 14 from the parous group were successful in nursing their babies for at least two months after delivery. The highest level of postpartum sexual interest in the first three months after delivery was reported by this group of nursing mothers. Not only did they report sexual stimulation (frequently to plateau tension levels and, on three occasions, to orgasm) induced by suckling their infants, but as a group they also described interest in as rapid return as possible to active coition with their husbands. There was a heavy overlay of guilt expressed by 6 of the 24 women who admittedly were

stimulated sexually by the suckling process. They were anxious to relieve concepts or fears of perverted sexual interest by reconstituting their normal marital relationships as quickly as possible. This concept has been reported previously and is only confirmed by this investigation.....

Fifty-eight of the 101 women reviewed during the postpartum period reported concern for their husbands' sexual tensions during the postpartum period of continence. Particularly were they concerned when postpartum continence was added to whatever pre-delivery-continence period had been established. Those women that had provided active relief for their husbands during third-trimester continence periods did so again after delivery. Three women in the parous and one in the previously nulliparous group had not approached their husbands before delivery, but during the postpartum period they assumed an active role in providing release for these men.

With the exception of the women for whom intercourse was interdicted medically for three months and the members of the nonmarried group, all women interviewed returned to full coital activity within six weeks to two months after delivery. Despite the fact that intercourse was prohibited for at least six weeks by most medical authorities, there frequently was return to coital activity within three weeks of delivery by higher-tensioned women or by wives attempting to respond to male demand. Particularly was an early return to coition the pattern for those women actively nursing (20).

The Masters and Johnson finding on the interest in earlier return to coition among breastfeeding women has often been repeated, often with the inference that this earlier return suggested an increased libido as compared with bottle-feeding women. The inference, however, seems to be at odds with clinical reports of numerous lactating women, who described a diminished libido during early lactation. This common lower level of sexual desire has also been noted by many writers on lactation (21,22,23,24,25,26,27).

An explanation for the earlier desire to resume coition by some women has been suggested that the women in the studies who chose to nurse tended to be women who felt more comfortable about using their bodies in an intimate relationship (27). If this postulate is true, as others have agreed, the cause and effect relationship between breastfeeding and the early return to coition may have been confused.

Cause	*Effects*
Being comfortable about using one's body in an intimate relationship.	1. Desire to breastfeed. 2. Earlier return to coition.

Thus, to suggest to the expectant father that breastfeeding will cause his wife to be more interested in returning to coition is misleading and possibly may lead to future disappointment.

Postpartum women, whether breast- or bottle feeding, may note less vaginal lubrication, which appears to be related to lower estrogen levels postpartum. This condition may cause intercourse to be painful. It often lasts longer in lactating women.

The effect of different styles of nursing on hormone levels, on the return of fertility, and on levels of sexual desire have been little investigated, but cannot be overlooked. Breastfeeding women who wean at 4 or 6 months, as did the only 3 nursing women actually studied by Masters and Johnson, may present a different pattern from women who nurse frequently, day and night, for an extended period of time. This is especially likely to be noticed in later months. For some nursing women lesser amounts of vaginal lubrication continue, along with lactational amenorrhea, for a year or more. Although a decreased level of sexual interest may no longer be noted after the tiredness and stress of early parenthood are diminished, the need for additional vaginal lubrication may continue for several months or for a year or more.

The lower level of sexual desire, although relatively common, is not universal. Sexual problems may be a symptom of poor communication and not be the cause of disharmony so much as the by-product (28). Couples whose sexual relationship was particularly satisfying before parturition are less likely to have problems postpartum. A woman who had no episiotomy or perineal tears is more likely to find sex comfortable early postpartum than a woman with an episiotomy repair or cesarean incision. Even when the episiotomy is well healed, the perineum may be tender but perhaps even more significant is the fact that the perineum has become associated with pain in the mind of the woman. It is understandable that the physical and emotional tiredness and stress that accompany adjusting to motherhood and fatherhood may strain sexual relations.

The nursing relationship of mother and baby may satisfy within the mother some of the needs that might otherwise have been satisfied by intercourse—feelings of closeness, fulfillment, and a reassurance that she is wanted and needed. Also, lactation by itself is an aspect of female sexuality, although it often is overlooked as such (21,29). Newton has pointed out that Kinsey's huge volume *Sexual Behavior of the Human Female* concentrated on only those portions of women's sexual behavior that are similar to what men experience (orgasm and coitis), while largely ignoring other important parts of women's sexuality such as lactation. She further pointed out that this discrepancy was seldom, if at all, noticed by reviewers of the book, whose habits of thought were in keeping with most of the culture (21).

There is deep physical pleasure involved in successful lactation. It is not surprising that, given the hormonal status, the fatique and stress in adjusting to parenthood, and the physical pleasure in nursing, that some postpartum lactating women temporarily feel compliant but not eager for sexual relations. However many advantages there are to breastfeeding, increasing the libido is *not* one of them.

Because the lower sex drive and lesser amount of vaginal lubrication do not seem advantageous and because it is often easier to avoid talking about sexual matters, such aspects of early lactation have not been widely publicized. Thus women must discover for themselves that they are less interested in sex than before the baby was born. Some women not aware of the transiency of the problem have feared that they have become permanently frigid. Knowing that the situation is normal, and transient, and that it is not "all in my head," is very reassuring.

The response of breastfeeding women may not be the main issue. How do bottle-feeding women feel about sex? Continuing to phrase the Masters and Johnson finding as it is usually quoted (Nursing women are *more* interested than non-nursing women.) emphasizes the contrast: it is the breast-feeders versus the bottle-feeders. This detracts from the larger issue of how postpartum women in general feel about sexuality, although generalizations may be difficult to make accurately. Of the 101 women interviewed in the third month postpartum by Masters and Johnson, 24 were breastfeeding, 77 bottle-feeding. All of the breastfeeding women were in the group reporting varying levels of sexual interest. But the other group (47 of the 101 women, apparently all bottle-feeding) described low or essentially negligible levels of sexuality. It would appear that a low libido is common among postpartum women in general.

Resumption of Intercourse Postpartum

Intercourse is permitted increasingly early in the postpartum period. This may not necessarily be welcome news to a woman, even when she realizes that there is no medical reason to recommend abstinence. A young wife who does not feel ready may feel that she is being pressured to engage in intercourse as a wifely duty. Also, it has been pointed out that a physician's statement to the effect that there is no reason for further abstinence may be misconstrued as a "command to perform," and if so, may be accompanied by increased anxiety on the part of either the man or woman (28).

As part of the advice given about the resumption of sexual relations, it is helpful to suggest that the woman use some form of addition lubrication, such as K-Y Sterile Lubricant. The initial act of intercourse is likely to be somewhat uncomfortable, especially for the woman who has had an episiotomy, but perhaps no more so at 3-4 weeks than it would be at 6-8 weeks.

The Postpartum Check-Up

There appear to be built-in dilemmas in helping the new parents who need help with sexual adjustment. Problems are likely to be particularly bothersome during the time period between 1 month and 6 months postpartum when the couple is not likely to be in contact with the physician. Even when a new mother and/or father has a concern about postpartum sexuality, they may hesitate to bring up the concern or make an appointment to discuss it. At the regular postpartum check-up, when the woman may not have yet engaged in coition, the concern may not be on her mind. Time limitations at the check-up increase the likelihood that other concerns take precedence.

The obstetrician, family practitioner or midwife who sees the woman for the routine postpartum check-up can discuss postpartum sexual relations. The importance of communication of feelings and needs between man and woman can be stressed. The woman can be reassured that decreased interest in sex postpartum is common, normal and transient. The need for additional lubrication may continue for prolonged periods in the breastfeeding woman.

Couples may have concerns that are a barrier to full enjoyment of sex because they hesitate to voice them, such as whether the lactating breasts are "off limits" (they are not).

Some women in early lactation do not enjoy having their breasts used in sexual foreplay; they may have tender breasts or sore nipples. Some, but not all, men do not enjoy stroking the firm breasts that are often characteristic of early lactation. If so, the couple may need to find new areas of the woman's body for sexual foreplay. Lactating breasts may also be relatively desensitized.

Couples react in different ways to the milk that leaks or sprays from the breasts at the time of orgasm. Most, but not all, women lose milk at this time. If the spraying milk is objectionable to either the woman or man (although he could interpret it as a positive sign of response), the loss of milk can be minimized by making love after a nursing when the breasts are relatively empty.

Some couples may fall into the mistaken assumption that there are only two choices: having sexual intercourse or lying on opposite sides of the bed. During the first month postpartum, a woman who feels this way may withdraw to her own side of the bed if she feels unready for or afraid of resuming coition. This may become a difficult pattern to break; the man may become afraid of making advances, afraid that he will be rejected. The nighttime separation can spiral and lead to the couple feeling more and more apart. Instead of thinking of loving in terms of sexual intercourse only especially in the first month postpartum, couples can be advised to use other ways of physical loving that are especially appropriate right after childbirth: holding, cuddling, giving back rubs, massage, fondling, sex play to orgasm. A lot of cuddling and fondling in the early weeks may make a return to coition seem more natural and relaxed.

LACTATING WOMEN IN SPECIAL SITUATIONS

As breastfeeding increases in popularity it is more and more difficult to characterize the "typical" breastfeeding mother. There are women in special situations who want to nurse and who may need specific extra help to ensure success. Many women in these situations would not have nursed even in the recent past.

Working Nursing Mothers

The working mother has become increasingly common. The trend back to breastfeeding has included both women who must and women who want to work outside the home. Increasingly, maternity leave is extended to up to 6 months, although women who need to work for financial reasons often must return sooner. A mother wishing to breastfeed should be encouraged to take full maternity leave privileges. If she does have 6 months, she can nurse her infant without worry about his nutritional needs when she does go back to work. By 6 months, babies can take fluids by cup and are beginning to be interested in solids. Ideally she can try to arrange to nurse him at a mid-day break, but even without this, her baby can learn to do without nursing through a full day's shift. Many babies will then nurse more often in the evening or night. Some find this extra time together after work very important compensation for being separated all day; others find frequent nursing after work difficult and prefer to wean, at this point, to a bottle.

If mother must go back to work at or before 3 to 4 months, she will need to consider either supplements of formula or expressed breastmilk or both. Some women express milk while they are at work and store it in a refrigerator to be given the next day by the baby sitter. Care must be taken in keeping the milk clean and refrigerated. Sterile disposable plastic bottle liners often are used. If mother and baby have been fully nursing for three months prior to the return to work, she may eventually be able to go without hand- or pump-expression during working hours without discomfort, the infant receiving formula for those missed feedings. Again, some nursing couples begin to increase night and evening nursings to compensate for the long period apart during the day while others prefer to wean or partially wean.

Breastfeeding a baby younger than 6 months while working full-time may not be easy. Women who are planning to return to work should be given not only practical pointers but also realistic advice. Although some working mothers continue to nurse happily for months, others find that their milk supply dwindles as the baby begins to prefer the bottle; this is especially likely for babies in the distractible 4 to 6 month age range. Expressing or pumping to provide enough milk for the next day's feedings is time-consuming and requires true commitment.

Hand expressing for comfort and possibly to prevent leaking may be necessary in the first few days back at work, even for the mother who does not want to collect milk. The milk supply soon adjusts, however, as less milk is removed from the breasts. Some women who begin by collecting enough milk for the next day's feedings decide that it is too time-consuming and discouraging and not worthwhile if the baby thrives on formula. In some such cases, when the mother only nurses before and after work, she may be disappointed as her milk supply dwindles. The combination of the dwindling milk supply and preference of some babies for the bottle makes continued nursing difficult after the first month of full-time working and nursing. If early weaning becomes inevitable, satisfaction in the early weeks of nursing should be looked back upon with pleasure and not be marred by disappointed feelings.

Other women continue to work and nurse very happily. Those women who successfully express or pump large amounts of milk for many weeks or months have a high level of commitment and find satisfaction from providing the milk for the time away from the baby.

Ideally, the working mother and baby enjoy a leisurely and loving nursing at the end of each working day, and before work. Realistically, this is not always possible in the early morning rush, or at the end of a busy day. The father's commitment to the child's nursing becomes critical. Giving a working mother adequate time to cuddle and nurse a 3-month-old by helping with older children and dinner may be vital to continued nursing.

Fearing to begin nursing because of a desire or need to return to work is unfounded. A young infant is easily weaned and whatever time that may have been spent nursing is valuable to both mother and infant.

The following points about working and nursing can be considered:

. . . . Tips for Counseling the Lactating Working Mother . . . .

1. Part-time work is usually more compatible with nursing than is full-time work especially for younger infants. Working close by to the baby can allow a midday nursing, which can help to maintain the milk supply and ease the separation of being apart. Some women have gone to where the baby is, or have the baby brought to them for nursing.

2. A mother can arrange with the sitter not to feed the young baby right before the time she will arrive to get him, making it more likely that the baby will nurse when she arrives.

3.   Has she accustomed the baby to the bottle? If she intends to use breast milk, an adequate supply should be in the freezer to compensate for days when she is unable to pump or express enough. Is she proficient at hand expression, or has she considered buying a small breast pump, such as the Kaneson or the Loyd-B? In many cases, it is wise to have on hand a supply of formula that is well tolerated by the baby.

4.   Some nursing couples begin to increase night and evening nursings to compensate for the long period apart during the day. Does this mother want to do this? Does she want to sleep with the baby in bed with her to encourage night nursings? It also is one way of ensuring continued high production of milk. This method is used by women in some foreign countries but does not appeal to most Western women.

5.   Does the mother want to try to nurse with no or few bottles on the days when she is not working? Some women, who express milk at work, are able to nurse on weekends without supplemental formula and have full breasts on Monday morning. Other women find that their milk supply is dwindling and weekend nursings are not enough to totally eliminate bottles of formula during the day on weekends.
    The continuing path of nursing is difficult to predict. How the baby reacts to nursing only before and after work may depend on his age when the mother returns to work, his disposition, how much time the mother has for nursing, and other factors. Some nursing couples continue to enjoy nursing for many months after the return to work.

6.   In many countries, there is nursing break legislation which guarantees a working nursing mother the time during her working day to nurse her infant (30). Provisions are made for day care close to work. Women are not penalized for time spent on breaks. Certainly such legislation in this country or voluntary commitment of private industries and businesses to this kind of arrangement would be beneficial to mothers and children. Young women often reach peak skill at a job and must then retire during the period of early child rearing. This system could make it more attractive for women to return to jobs.
    Presently, nursing during the working day is still the exception. Most working mothers are separated from their infants for many hours, and they require information on how to manage. Most of the practical information on managing breastfeeding for working mothers is the same as for other

mothers. Getting a baby accustomed to a bottle is the same. The information on storing and/or defrosting breast milk is the same. (See Chapter 14)

The Ghetto Mother

Problems of malnutrition and increased infant morbidity and mortality among the urban poor are well publicized. The advantages of breastfeeding (nutritional, immunological, psychological, and of economy) make it an obvious choice for the urban poor. Unfortunately, the factors needed to encourage successful lactation are most often lacking in this setting. Improved health care programs for expectant mothers and children could include better education in health matters, specifically, information about nutrition and breastfeeding (31).

The Mother with a Chronic Disease or Handicap

Mothers with many of the medical disorders can be advised that nursing is possible for them. In some cases it may be easier than formula feeding and may give the women much pleasure. The limiting factor in many cases will be maternal medications required and the lack of safety of them for the nursing newborn. (See Chapter 3) In some cases the acuteness of the mother's illness and her ability to care for her infant physically may also be a factor. Perhaps one of the most common chronic diseases is diabetes mellitus where clearly nursing can be successful. The mother may need extra help in maintaining a diet sufficient to meet her extra nutritional needs and in helping to determine an appropriate adjustment of her insulin dosage.

The woman with a physical handicap such as blindness or motor handicap such as paraplegia may profit from the special advantages of ease and constant availability that nursing brings.

The Mother Who is Hospitalized

At times a nursing couple faces separation because of maternal illness. Obviously if mother is seriously ill, abrupt weaning may be necessary. Often, however, the hospitalization is brief. In such cases, she needs special help in maintaining her milk supply and in arranging to nurse her infant as often and as soon as possible. Most often the woman's family finds it necessary to rent or acquire a pump. This should be arranged as soon as possible. (Many maternity units will not lend pumps to other units in the same hospital.) The mother may need help in learning how to use the pump and in the actual physical effort. The importance of early and frequent expressing of breast milk cannot be overemphasized. Engorged breasts are painful, at high risk for infection and make efficient pumping very difficult.

As soon as the mother's condition permits, the nursing baby can be brought to her. Special arrangements may be necessary to satisfy hospital rules but are greatly appreciated by the mother and are worthwhile. Bringing the mother to a quiet lobby or other area where infants are allowed, or perhaps to an area in the pediatric wing, are possible alternatives. Cooperation of several medical services may be needed.

References

1. Lloyd, JK: Chairman's Introduction. CIBA Foundation Symposium 45:1, 1976.

2. Jelliffe, EFP: Maternal nutrition and lactation. CIBA Foundation Symposium 45:119, 1976.

3. Higginbottom, MC et al: A syndrome of methylmalonic aciduria, homocystinuria, megalobastic anemia and neurologic abnormalities in a vitamin B-12 deficient breast-fed infant of a strict vegetarian, New Engl. J. Med. 299:317, 1978.

4. Binkiewicz, A et al: Pseudo-Cushing syndrome caused by alcohol in breast milk, J. Pediatr. 93:965, 1978.

5. American Academy of Pediatrics Committee on Environmental Hazards, PCBs in Breast Milk. 62:407, 1978.

6. Lappé, FM: *Diet for a Small Planet.* New York: Ballantine Books, 1971.

7. U. S. Medicine, July 15, 1978.

8. Knodel, J: Breast-feeding and population growth, Science 198:1111, 1977.

9. Tyson, JE et al: Significance of the secretion of human prolactin and gonadotropin for puerperal lactational infertility. CIBA Foundation Symposium 45:49, 1976.

10. Kippley, S: *Breast-Feeding and Natural Child Spacing.* New York: Penguin Books, 1974.

11. Van Ginneken, JK: The Chance of Conception during Lactation from Fertility Regulation during Human Lactation. (Parks, AS et al, eds.) Cambridge, England: Galton Foundation, 1977.

12. Brunner, DL et al: Prolactin levels in nursing mothers, Am. J. Obstet. Gynecol. 131:250, 1978.

13. Meara, H: A key to successful breastfeeding in a non-supportive culture, J. of Nurse-Midwifery 21 (1), 1976.

14. Nursing Mothers Committee of the Childbirth Education Association of Greater Philadelphia.

15. Ebrahim, GJ: Cross cultural aspects of breastfeeding - CIBA Foundation symposium 45:195, 1976.

16. Savena, PC: Breastfeeding: its effects on postpartum amenorrhea. Social Biology 24:45, 1971.

17. Avery, JL: *Induced Lactation: A Guide for Counseling and Management.* Denver: J. J. Avery, Inc., 1972.

18. Billings, J: *Natural Family Planning- The Ovulation Method.* Collegeville, MN: The Liturgical Press, 1972.

19. Kavanagh-Jazrawy, F, ed.: *Planning Your Family the Sympto-Thermal Way.* Ottawa, Ontario: Sereina Canada, 1975.

20. Masters, W and Johnson, V: *Human Sexual Response.* Boston: Little, Brown & Co., 1966.

21. Newton, N: *Maternal Emotions.* New York: Paul B. Hoeber, Inc., 1955.

22. Gunther, M: The New Mother's View of Herself. CIBA Foundation Symposium 45:152, 1976.

23. Bricklin, AG: *Mother Love.* Philadelphia: Running Press, 1975.

24. Pryor, K: *Nursing Your Baby.* New York: Pocket Book Division of Simon & Schuster, 1973.

25. Ewy, D and R: *Preparation for Breast Feeding.* New York: Dolphin Books, 1975.

26. The Boston Women's Health Book Collective. *Our Bodies, Ourselves.* New York: Simon & Schuster, 1976.

27. Bing, E and Colman, L: *Making Love During Pregnancy.* Bantam, 1977.

28. Greenberg, M and Brenner, P: The newborn's impact on parents' marital and sexual relationship, Medical Aspects of Human Sexuality : 16, 1977.

29. Francis, B: Successful lactation and women's sexuality, J. Trop. Pediatr. 22 (4), Aug. 1976.

30. Richardson, JL: Legislation regarding nursing breaks, J. Trop. Pediatr. 21:249, 1975.

31. Jenkins, ME, ed., *Child Health in the Ghetto: Infant Mortality and Morbidity.* Washington, D. C.: Howard University.

Chapter 12

The Continuing
Course of Normal Lactation

AGES AND STAGES

Breastfeeding is described in this chapter as it changes from infancy through three and four years of age. Although nursing is considered to be appropriate only for infants in most of the Western world, nursing continues for several years in many cultures, averaging two to three years.

The nursing relationship changes as the child grows. The frequent, long nursings and full leaking breasts characteristic of the early months of nursing are very different from the often brief occasional "snack" of the two-year-old.

Rarely is breastfeeding behavior a matter of the baby's behavior alone. It is the interaction between the two members of the team, whether at two days postpartum, or at two years. The baby acts and the mother reacts.

This chapter will address itself to the types of questions that mothers ask which are relevant mostly to one of the several stages of human development.

The stages have been divided according to different characteristic breastfeeding behaviors, somewhat arbitrarily, as follows:

1.   the newborn: birth to 3 months

2.   the middle-aged infant: approximately 4 to 7 months

3.   the older infant: approximately 8 to 12 months

4.   the young toddler: approximately 12 to 18 or 20 months

5.   the older toddler: nursing from 1½ to 2 years up to 3 or
4 years.

Birth to Three Months

Breastfeeding means both food and comfort. There are many books and
many theories which seek to give us insight into the newborn period. Selma
Fraiberg offers some insight into the study of newborn infants:

> The psychologist, too, has trouble in getting this fellow to
> reveal his inner life. He is the most uncooperative of all
> subjects. His close-mouthed attitude toward the researcher
> is responsible for a great deal of scientific dissension in the
> field of early infancy and for extraordinary flights of scien-
> tific imagination as well. In any case, the subject of these
> investigations does not engage in controversy and some of
> the most extravagant and daring theories of the inner life of
> infancy have never been disproved. Neither have they been
> proved.
>   We are probably on safe ground with the infant if we
> begin with few assumptions and work with the meager in-
> formation that can be gained through direct observation. We
> see very little in the first two months that we call "mental."
> In these early weeks the infant functions on the basis of need
> and satisfaction. His hunger is a ravenous hunger, the tensions
> it produces are intolerable, and the satisfaction of this hunger
> is imperative . (1)

The baby reacts to all discomforts—hunger, gas pains, loneliness, bore
dom—by crying. The baby has no conception that he and his mother are
separate individuals, and so there is no fear or anxiety at being separated. In
fact, the baby may calm down and stop crying when he is taken from the
arms of a tense mother and held by someone who is calm.

One theory on infancy relates well to counseling new breastfeeding
mothers. It has been said that finding trust is what is basic to the newborn
baby. If the baby's needs are met in early infancy, he will develop a sense of
trust, trust in his mother and trust that the world is a good and caring place
Many questions that new mothers ask involve a fear that they will spoil the
baby and can be answered by helping the mothers to realize that their
babies, in the first month or two of life, need to develop this sense of trust
They do not need to be shown that the parents are in control, as is implied
by such questions as "Should I pick him up every time he cries?" "Is it a
good idea to nurse him as often as he seems to want to?" Parents who under
stand the feelings and needs of young infants will find an understanding of
breastfeeding easier. If the mother wants her baby to trust the world, she

will not hesitate to nurse her baby as often as is needed, which may be 10 times in 24 hours.

All parents are individuals and all need to find their own style of parenting; often this is one of their tasks in the first month of their baby's life. The professional should not only help them learn the normal pattern of early breastfeeding but also help them to be comfortable with their own infant and with their style of parenting, by helping them to find their own answers. Some mothers, however, have definite opinions on child development that may make successful breastfeeding unlikely. If mother tries to show the baby that she is the boss, if she believes that hunger is the only real need in infancy, or if she follows rigid schedules, breastfeeding is likely to fail.

Nutrition

No supplemental foods are needed during this period. If the mother is well nourished and the baby full-term, there is need only for consideration of vitamin D and fluoride supplement. At present, vitamin D drops are available in combination with vitamins A and C, although these latter vitamins are not needed.

The 1979 recommendation of the American Academy of Pediatrics for fluoride supplements in the totally breastfed infant is 0.25 mg/day, regardless of the fluoride content in the drinking water (2). (Breast milk contains little fluoride even in areas of fluoridated water.)

Many new mothers are concerned about their baby's stool pattern. They may have never seen the loose yellow seedy stools of the breastfed infant and may be concerned about the frequency as well as the looseness of the baby's stools. Anywhere from one stool at every feeding (a stain on the diaper) to one every 7 or 8 days is normal for breastfed babies. This is neither diarrhea nor constipation and needs no treatment. Mothers ask about the color and may get concerned over any tinge of green. Stool color from green to yellow is normal. The color reflects variation in bowel transit time and is caused by bile salts. An occasional greenish stool in an otherwise well baby is normal. A pattern of passing scanty and infrequent stools may indicate that an infant is not receiving enough milk.

There may be changes in a baby's normal stool because of some change within the mother. A cracked, bleeding nipple may produce a trace of blood which the baby swallows as he nurses, causing a darker stool. Sometimes a mother may know that her nipple is sore, but not realize that it is bleeding, especially if the crack is on the bottom of the nipple. Medication can change the color and/or consistency of the baby's stool. Commonly when the mother is taking an antibiotic for a breast infection, the infant's stools become loose. Unless the mother understands that this is a reaction to the drug, she may fear that her milk is "germy" and has given the baby diarrhea.

Sleeping

The young baby's sleeping and nursing behaviors are part of a single pattern. A newborn may nurse 7-12 times in 24 hours and seem to be on no discernible schedule at all. Many babies have one longer sleep time of 4-6 hours and need to nurse every 1½-3 hours at other times. Most young babies fall asleep easily at the breast; a few fall asleep easily if left alone in the crib.

By three months many babies have settled into an approximate schedule or have a somewhat predictable pattern. The number of hours of sleep in a 24 hour period varies from 10 hours for those infants with low sleep requirements to 20 hours for others. Most babies' sleep needs are somewhere in between. Many mothers need to be reassured that their baby's pattern is normal, although not necessarily "average." Often babies take several "cat naps," which help to fulfill their sleep requirements. Unfortunately from the mother's point of view, these naps do not allow the mother enough time to nap herself or to get a feeling of accomplishment from doing other things.

Whether or not a baby sleeps through the night is a matter of definition. One mother will complain, "I wish he'd sleep through the night. He sleeps *only* from 12 to 5 in the morning." , while another mother will call that same 12 to 5 pattern "sleeping through the night." Some babies sleep 6 to 8 hours from the time they are a week old. Many do not, but gradually stretch out the length of time that they sleep. Many young babies nurse one or two or more times/night. A mother may find that she can cope with her baby's need to nurse at night if she can keep the baby's bassinet or car bed next to her bed and just reach over and pick up the baby to nurse. A second woman does not want the baby in the same room with her. A third woman sleeps with the baby in bed with her all night.

There is no guaranteed solution for curing night wakefulness. Mothers ask if cereal or a bottle or letting the baby cry it out would help. These solutions have sometimes resulted in an individual baby sleeping longer, but often have had no effect. Some babies have reacted to the cereal or bottle of cows' milk formula by spitting up or having a reaction that makes their sleep worse. Some babies cry briefly and then go to sleep; other babies will cry until they are frantic and no one in the house gets any sleep at all.

It may help to advise the mother not to awaken herself fully for the middle of the night feedings, so that she is able to go back to sleep when the baby does. With a first baby especially, the mother may have never before had to learn how to go back to sleep after being awakened. The new mother can be advised not to change diapers in the middle of the night. Naps by mothers during the day can be encouraged.

Reaction of the Culture to the Breastfeeding Couple

The mother is praised by many people for nursing her baby. Those who are not personally familiar with breastfeeding think in terms of the physical advantages to the baby. They assume that this is why the woman is nursing. The woman's own feelings may range from enjoying the closeness, to inner doubts about her ability to provide enough milk, enough mothering, enough love. Some degree of postpartum depression is not unusual. During pregnancy everyone asked about the mother, but now all questions and interest are focused on the baby.

Suggestions

The mother needs reassurance. What the nursing mother of a new baby also needs is time to adjust and help in differentiating parenting problems from breastfeeding problems (see also Chapter 9).

The Middle-Aged Infant (approximately 4-7 months)

Breastfeeding continues for many nursing couples beyond the first three or four months. Those women who choose to continue are generally, but not always, thought well of for doing more than "getting him off to a good start." It is the infant's behavior change at the breast that makes many women question whether or not they should continue. The middle-aged infant is so distracted and distractable at the breast that he sometimes makes the mother feel unappreciated. The mother who enjoyed nursing her young baby for many peaceful hours may need to be told that she can expect this change. The baby can't help but look around the room—even while he is nursing. Anyone or anything distracts him. Mothers who do not understand that this change is normal often feel that breastfeeding is no longer important and wonder if they should wean. Often taking the child to a quieter place may help keep his attention during a feeding.

There is a second difference between young and middle-aged nursing babies: the older baby is so *efficient* at the breast that he can empty both sides in just a few minutes. He can get a lot of milk in a very short time. Again, the problem is the mother's unfamiliarity with the normal pattern of breastfeeding after 4 months of age. The mother who does not realize how much milk he is getting may wonder whether the nursing is worth doing or worry that her supply is dwindling—and again think about weaning.

Another possible problem is the baby's *teething behavior*. If his gums are sore he may not want to nurse for very long, although this is not true for all babies; some seem to want to nurse longer and more often during teething.

It has been suggested that teething is not responsible for all that is blamed on it. Normal periods of "fussing," which cannot be blamed on any discernible cause, are often said to be due to teething. Separation anxiety happens at about the same time as the first teeth come in, and it is not always possible to know for which reason a baby is crying. "He must be teething!" is a convenient phrase to use because it doesn't place blame on anyone. It also depicts the cause as a physical, rather than an emotional one.

The other big concern about teeth centers on the "Suppose he bites me" question. Some mothers assume that they will need to wean when the teeth appear because they have not been told otherwise. It is helpful to reassure the mother of a baby who does not yet have teeth that when the first lower teeth appear, they will be covered by the tongue when the baby is nursing. The mother can be reassured by noticing the tip of the baby's tongue, which she can see up against the lower part of her nipple. But what about the upper teeth? It might seem that there is nothing to protect the nipple from them. Yet with the baby's mouth in the nursing position, the teeth cannot generally be felt.

Some mothers have heard stories about babies deliberately biting and they may wonder: "When is this going to happen to me?" The answer is that some babies never bite; for those who do bite, the problem is a manageable one. Most often the baby is predictable. He clamps down near the end of a nursing or acts playful before trying to bite. Some babies bite only once or twice in many months of nursing. They can and do learn not to bite.

The following are suggestions to give to the mother whose baby has bitten her:

. . . . Measures Against Biting. . . . .

1. Advise her to give the teething baby lots of other things to teethe on. A cold washcloth before nursing can soothe his gums.

2. Tell the mother to watch for a change in the baby's nursing pattern. After the period of fast nursing action by the baby's mouth and his fast swallowing is over, the mother whose baby is a biter can stop the feeding. She can break suction, and if the baby is hungry, she can nurse him on the other side. She should never continue to nurse when the baby is acting playful.

3. Suggest that the mother keep a finger handy next to the baby's mouth to be ready to break suction quickly if the baby gets a playful look in his eye, or if the baby's mouth action changes to a chewing type of mouth action.

4. If the baby does bite down, the mother should, and undoubtedly will, say "NO!" and stop the feeding. Some women may need to be helped not to feel guilty about "yelling" at the baby. Others may need to be counseled not to overdo the yelling and thus frighten the baby so that he refuses to nurse at all.

Nutrition

The appearance of teeth at around six months is a clue that the baby is getting ready for solids. Nutritionally, the baby of a well nourished mother does not need any food other than breast milk until the middle of the first year. The well full-term-infant can triple his birth weight without requiring supplemental iron, if the maternal iron status is normal. Premature babies, babies born to mothers with severe iron deficiency in pregnancy, or babies with some other source of blood loss often will need additional iron before six months of age.

Once solids are added, iron will then be obtained from the solids he receives. Iron fortified cereals and meats are good sources of iron during this period.

Vitamin D supplementation can be continued for the breastfed infant, particularly if there is little exposure to sunlight. 0.25 mg/day of fluoride can be continued as long as the child is totally breastfed. Fluoride dose should then be decreased in areas of natural fluoridation or appropriately adjusted once solids are taken regularly.

During this period the baby is beginning to explore his environment. He reaches for objects and puts almost everything in his mouth. He is developmentally ready for finger foods. Which first foods and the order of foods introduced are a matter of personal preference. Helping mothers to begin feeding solids should include reassurance that it is a gradual process and that babies' tastes vary.

Sleeping

Some middle-aged infants have always slept through the night. Others still do not. Some babies were sleeping through but begin to awaken one time or more. In the latter case, the explanation may be hunger. A baby who is very distracted in the daytime may nurse only briefly and may not be stimulating his mother's milk supply to remain copious. This is more likely to happen with a second or third baby: the prime offenders in the "distractor" category are older siblings. If a baby seems actually to be hungry at night, or if a baby who used to sleep through the night now begins to awaken, the mother needs to make a conscious effort to increase the number of calories he gets from the breast milk in the daytime. This involves nursing away from all distractions whenever possible.

As mentioned before, another commonly suggested reason for a baby to begin to awaken at night is pain from teething. Whether or not this is the cause on a particular night is difficult to determine. Some babies just seem to want company and the comfort of nursing, at night.

Most middle-aged babies do have predictable periods of sleeping and waking in the day and night. Often they have a morning and an afternoon nap. The mothers of babies who do not respond to their attempts to have them sleep at predictable times may need help in accepting a situation which they do not like. Other mothers do not seem to mind not knowing when their babies are going to sleep or nurse. All patterns are "normal."

The mother of a baby who has never slept through the night may (or may not) be reassured to hear that most old baby books expected babies to have night feedings. Older books also recommended that the mother take a fussy baby to bed with her.

The question of whether or not a mother *ought* to sleep with her baby in bed with her may be asked. Sleeping together is compatible with breast-feeding. Its roots are old and with historical and cultural basis (3). Whether or not sleeping with the baby is a good idea or a terrible one is in the realm of opinion, not fact, and must be each family's own decision.

A mother who feels most comfortable with the baby near her can be encouraged to take the baby into bed *if* that is what she seems to want to do or already has been doing it. The loss of privacy may make the idea unacceptable to some parents. Others find it an answer to nighttime problems. The mother of a very young infant may feel safer keeping the child in a cot or in a nearby crib, taking the baby into bed only for feedings and keeping him only long enough for him to fall back to sleep.

Coping with Distraction
. . . . .in the Middle-Aged Infant. . . . .

1.   Suggest that the mother nurse in a quiet, fairly dark room. She may plan to nurse while her older child is occupied watching TV or visiting a neighbor or napping, whenever possible. Some distracted babies will nurse happily if their mothers turn so that they can nurse and watch the action at the same time. Some babies resume nursing if their mothers allow them some play time when they seem to want it during a feeding.

2.   Some mothers of very distractable babies find that their babies nurse best in the dark.

3.   Help the mother to understand her baby's efficiency at the breast—while still encouraging her to let the baby nurse

for longer stretches when he is willing, such as when he is sleepy. This will better maintain her milk supply.

4.   Reassure the mother that nursing is still very important to the baby despite his casual attitude. The baby feels comfortable in playing at the breast because he has learned to feel sure that he can enjoy the security of nursing.

The Older Infant (approximately 7 or 8 to 12 months)

In the Western countries the last part of the first year is the traditional time to wean, although the average age for weaning for much of the world is between 2 and 3 years. One reason the Western countries consider weaning between 7 and 12 months to be appropriate is because of the behavior of many babies. Many go through what may be called a "learning spurt" around nine months. The older baby is interested in exploring the world by crawling, by beginning to walk and by exploring his environment. The baby feels comfortable doing all this exploring so long as he can go back to his mother as a safe home base. The baby not only crawls back, but searches the room with his eyes to be sure his mother is there. It is understandable from the baby's point of view that he would like to have her always in sight, but this can be hard on the mother's patience. The baby often whimpers or howls whenever the mother leaves the room. Some women find it easier to carry the baby with them when they go to the bathroom, rather than have to soothe the baby's feelings of abandonment. The two typical behaviors of this age—the crawling away, and the checking back for reassurance—are found in all babies, but one or the other behavior often seems to be dominant in a particular baby What does all this have to do with breastfeeding?

It is the crawling away, the interest in new things, that leads people to assume that weaning is in order. The baby seems to be so "grown up;" he can manage solid food from a cup and spoon. On many days the baby is too busy to ask to nurse as he once used to. When the mother picks up the baby and offers the breast, he may seem not to be interested. For many babies, nine months is an easy time to wean. Mothers who find the idea of nursing a toddler unappealing should definitely be urged to take advantage of this situation to wean. It is not as easy in many cases to wean a toddler or child.

There are other babies whose emphasis is on the checking back for reassurance. They prefer to do most of their exploring visually from the security of their mother's lap. Babies of this type do not give out the same signals of wanting to wean. They love to nurse and cuddle, but they can be weaned if the mother wants to wean them.

Somehow, discussion on the nursing of older babies often centers on weaning advice. But what about the mother who wants to continue to nurse? She is more likely to be a mother who has nursed a previous child, or who is in contact with a breastfeeding support group. What is nursing like with an eight- to twelve-month-old baby? Babies of this age enjoy food other than mother's milk. For the first time the benefit to the child in nursing switches somewhat from food to comfort. Some babies nurse for only a few minutes at a time and then climb down to explore again. Most have one or two longer nursings, at nap or bedtime, or in the early morning.

Women who have nursed older babies usually list the main advantage to be the surefire ability to *comfort* a sick or fussy baby while providing excellent nutrition at the same time. The advice to "encourage fluids" which is frequently given to the mother of an ill child doesn't come close in terms of nutrition or comfort. Women who have had one baby already weaned by nine months and then go on to nurse the next child longer wonder how they made it with the first baby through the teething and illnesses and crying in the night without the longer period at the breast. Even when older babies are well, nursing has advantages over other ways of providing good nutrition, comfort, skin contact and touching. It's not that all these things can't be otherwise provided; it's just that nursing is an *easier* and *very complete* way of providing all at the same time.

Most women who have had personal experience with nursing an older baby are glad that they did. But there are some few women who are not so positive; while they would definitely nurse a subsequent baby, they would never continue nursing beyond eight or nine months. Yet most people who do have personal experience with nursing beyond two years encourage others to do so. Women who have nursed until their babies were two years old or older often have difficulty in understanding those who wean "early."

The decision of when to wean is not the physician's to make; it is a family decision. The appropriate role of the professional is to give accurate information to help make the decision the correct one for each nursing couple.

Nutrition

It is generally assumed that older babies receive only a small percentage of their total calories from breast milk. Some older babies, however, do receive a considerable number of calories from it.

A mother who is worried because her baby doesn't seem to want to eat very much can be reassured (if baby's weight gain is constant and adequate) to learn that older babies need comparatively smaller amounts of food than they did as infants. The mother also can be comforted by a reminder that breast milk is still an excellent food. The mother may also need to be reminded that the small amounts of food that her baby does eat should contain the additional nutrients that her baby most needs, especially iron. Women whose babies are not interested in solid food can be encouraged to offer the solids *before* nursing. A fussy or frantic baby may refuse all but the breast, however, until after he has nursed for a while.

Sleeping

It is generally assumed that all babies sleep through the night by the time they are eight months old. Many do, but many do awaken at least some nights. Often teething is said to be the cause. Again, teething often is mentioned because it is a physical cause that cannot be blamed on anyone—and it may well be the cause at times.

In some families, and in many cultures, babies are allowed to nurse through the night well into toddlerhood; the baby who awakens at night is simply nursed quietly back to sleep (see also the suggestions later in the chapter).

Young Toddler (approximately 12-18 months)

In most ways the nursing toddler is no different from any other toddler. He is walking and getting into everything. The fact that toddlers seem so grown up in motor development may be one reason why nursing seems to be inapproriate to most people in Western cultures. The main reason why nursing the toddler seems inappropriate is that it is an unfamiliar phenomenon in Western culture. Friends or relatives who know that the baby still is nursing may begin to question the mother's motivation, to themselves or aloud. "Why doesn't she wean that child?" It is thought that the mother will spoil the toddler or make him too dependent on her. Being criticized is something that no one likes, but being criticized for doing what seems to be right for one's child can hurt deeply. Even families who were totally supportive can begin to surprise the mother with "Wean now!" advice or sarcastic remarks.

Most women who are nursing a toddler need reassurance from someone, or at least from a book, that many other women have done the same thing. Getting to talk to someone else in the same situation can be a relief.

Nursing a toddler is very different from nursing a young baby. Many toddlers nurse for only a minute or two at a time during a busy day. The nursing is a brief, but effective way for the toddler to be reassured. The mother of a toddler is not nursing him for the same reasons that she nursed him as a newborn. She is nursing him because it is a comfort and because *both* members of the nursing couple enjoy it.

There are some toddlers who want to nurse ten times a day, if the mother will go along with this. Her attitude is probably, "If it keeps him happy, why not?" Some toddlers nurse erratically, ten times one day and none the next. This great fluctuation in demand can be a cause of mastitis in a very few women.

Nutrition
Toddlers, nursing or not, are sometimes known for eating only small amounts of food. Their mothers often worry because they eat much less than they did in the first year of life. After checking that the child's weight gain is adequate, mothers need to be told that this smaller appetite is normal. The small appetite of a nursing toddler is not being "ruined" by breast milk. Breast milk is still valuable nutritionally.

Sleeping
Some, but not all, toddlers still nurse to sleep before bed or naptime. Some accept more willingly than others being put to bed without nursing. Most will accept it happily if the mother is not home. The one point about toddler nursing that makes more women question the wisdom of what they are do-ing is the "sleeping through the night" issue. There are no controlled stud-ies, but experience seems to indicate that nursing toddlers do wake up more often at night, to nurse. Non-nursing toddlers awaken at night too, but not with as much regularity. Many nursing toddlers awaken more than once every night so that they can nurse. Some toddlers awaken five times a night to nurse. Few non-nursing toddlers awaken that many times a night.

What can be said to help a mother who finds herself getting up to nurse one or more times every night?

Suggestions for Night Awakenings
. . . . .in the Nursing Toddler . . . . ·

1.   The father can comfort the baby; he can offer a drink of water.

2.   The baby can be put to bed with an older sibling, if there is one.

3.   The mother may comfort the baby without nursing and thus make the nighttime attention seem less desirable.

4.   The baby can sleep on a padded area or a mattress on the floor. The mother can nurse him and slip away, leaving the baby undisturbed. (This is for those women who do not want to sleep with the baby.)

5. She can take the baby to her bed. It will make the night nursings less tiring. This probably should be the mother's own idea, but it can be given support by the professional as an alternative. The last two suggestions, however, will not discourage the baby from awakening to nurse.

There are two somewhat different points of view on the topic of toddlers awakening to nurse in the night. Most feel that nighttime awakening should be discouraged. The other school of thought defends the normalcy of "biological night feedings" (4). There is no proof that either view is correct or better than the other. Most people (medical and lay) have an opinion on this issue that influences their recommendations for handling the situation. When a mother says that her toddler is awakening at night, she may or may not be certain of how she and the father feel about the issue. The physician (or other health professional) who is a resource for parents, rather than a decision-maker, can mention the two schools of thought. Parents who need help in deciding how they feel about nighttime awakening may want to read Fraiberg: *The Magic Years* (which supports parents who want to stop the awakening), and Thevenin: *The Family Bed* (which is reassuring about the normalcy of nighttime awakening and of taking the child into bed with the parents; see the references at the end of this chapter).

The Older Toddler (Nursing children 2, 3, and 4 years old)
The idea of nursing an older child elicits a strongly negative emotional reaction from many people, but mainly from those who have no personal or family experience with it. The woman who chooses to nurse after 1½-2 years in Western countries is very aware that she is unusual. She may gain status or interest if she is a member or a leader in a breastfeeding support group, but, even so, she is likely to be criticized by others who know that she is still nursing. Many women and children who are nursing couples are "closet" nursers. Their friends, neighbors, relatives and pediatricians often do not know that the child is still nursing.

Some women who have thought ahead or who have been appropriately forewarned have taught the child to say: "I want night night," or "I want lovey," instead of saying, "I want to nurse." This ploy is often useful since most two and three year old children are neither reticent nor soft-spoken.

With nursing at this age, the children are verbally proficient. The mother can say, "Only upstairs in our nursing chair," or "We don't nurse in stores". Some women defend the nursing as the best part of mothering and resent feeling pressure to keep the fact a secret from others.

If the motivation of a woman nursing a young toddler is sometimes suspect, imagine the suspicions that a mother nursing a two or three year old arouses: Why is she doing it? Does she get a somewhat perverted thrill out of it? Doesn't she realize it isn't good for the boy or for the girl? Nursing a child that "old" seems to some to have a sexual connotation.

The nursing is for comfort and love, although breast milk is still a nutritious food for a two or three or four year old child. The mother's let-down takes longer, even a few minutes to function. The woman may not be aware of any let-down. There is less milk than there was earlier. On the other hand, a few children are so fond of sitting on their mother's lap to nurse that they do encourage a noticeable milk supply. Rarely they may even nurse so much that they have less appetite for other foods—and then advice on cutting back is appropriate. Most nursing children nurse for only a few minutes at a time and act the same as non-nursing children for the rest of the day. Many are the last child in a busy family, where there is always a lot of activity going on. The couple just keep nursing because they both enjoy those few peaceful minutes between the other daily activities.

Occasionally, however, a mother is nursing her child and trying to treat him like a baby because she doesn't know how else to mother him. She is stuck and needs to learn what else to do with a two or three year old. It may never have occurred to her to read him a picture book or take him for a walk to talk about what they see. Taking him to a park or to a play group or nursery school may be useful suggestions to make to the mother.

The feelings in retrospect of women who have nursed an older child are in general more positive than women who are in the middle of nursing one. Looking back on it, the experience seems to be positive and free from doubts. Of course it was the right thing to do. Look how well-adjusted and independent the child is now. Women who have nursed older children usually recommend it to other women. The women who are currently nursing a child often have some doubts along with the good feelings. "Is he really going to wean when he is ready? When?" Babyish behavior that *all* children display from time to time sometimes is attributed to the nursing, possibly by a father who had been supportive of nursing, up to the third year. Even women who feel very strongly in favor of the nursing of children get annoyed at the criticism.

Along with an occasional doubt on the mother's part, "Am I sure I want to keep nursing a three year old?", there is also another feeling. The mother knows that she now has two choices: to try to wean now, or to keep nursing for awhile. Knowing her child, she may feel that to keep nursing would be easier, less traumatic, and a more loving choice than weaning. She may be reassured that children in other countries often nurse for two or three or more years.

WEANING

In simple terms, weaning is the reverse of building up a milk supply. The baby nurses less, so the breasts produce less milk.

In "mother-led weaning", the mother makes the decision to wean her baby; this is the usual pattern in weaning young infants. In "baby-led weaning," the baby decides that he no longer wants to nurse, frequently at around nine months of age. In many cultures where nursing continues beyond infancy, it is usually tradition, or the adults, and not the child, who decide when and how to initiate weaning. Since weaning, like nursing, involves interaction and interpretation between both members of the nursing couple, the distinction between mother-led and baby-led weaning is sometimes difficult to make. The mother's interpretation of her child's behavior is likely to be a very strong determining factor in when and how weaning occurs. There is a tendency for first babies to "wean themselves" by the end of the first year, while subsequent babies tend to nurse longer. The last child—the baby—in a large family of breastfed children, is unlikely to wean before two years.

A first-time mother generally is thrilled by each sign of developmental progress: the first tooth, the first steps. She enjoys watching her baby grow up. Because she interprets what he is doing as "grown up" behavior, she stops offering the breast. Unconsciously she is encouraging weaning.

Another mother, one who has had several other children, knows how babyish two year olds can sometimes be and does not think of a 9-month-old baby as grown-up. If this is to be her last baby, she may not want to think of this child as growing up too quickly. The baby may exhibit identical behavior as the baby of the first-time mother, but because she prefers to think of him as a baby, she continues to offer the breast regularly and so unconsciously she is encouraging continued nursing.

Women are not always conscious of the way in which they encourage either weaning or continued nursing. The two women mentioned above will not request the same weaning advice.

If babies are allowed to continue nursing beyond the first year, they often will continue nursing well into the second year, longer if allowed. Children sometimes wean themselves at 18 or 24 months, but many do not. After about 18 months, the child's awareness of his part in nursing makes him a more controlling member of the nursing couple. A two year old may cuddle, read books, agree to skip a nursing and wean happily, but on the other hand he may object. Weaning a two year old who would rather nurse is not easy. The mother who finds toddler nursing unappealing is best advised to initiate weaning by the end of the first year. The mother who waits for her child to take the lead in weaning may be waiting for some time!

Some women with young babies believe that weaning will solve commonly encountered baby problems such as fussing, colic and nighttime wakefulness, while others have a vague hope that things will somehow be better after weaning. Perhaps the most common concern among new mothers is a nagging fear that the baby's (normal) episodes of crying are caused by an inadequate milk supply. But weaning does not make babies stop having a fussy time, nor does it make babies sleep through the night. Weaning does not make mothers feel young again. Thus it is often appropriate for the professional to help the woman to clarify her expectations about weaning.

There are two main steps in the weaning process, whether the child is two weeks or three years old. These two steps are *substituting* something else for each nursing and *watching* for any physical or emotional reactions in the child or mother.

1. Each mother should be advised to think in terms of substituting for each nursing, not of eliminating nursings (or "dropping" or "skipping" them). The substitute should ideally be just as good as nursing from the baby's point of view. For a young baby, a good substitute is cuddling him while offering a bottle of formula. For an older baby, a good substitute might be a cup of apple juice and looking at a picture book with his mother.

2. The second step—watching for any reactions—should help the mother in managing the weaning process.

The weaning process is a matter of continuing with the two steps until no more nursings remain. The process may be completed fairly rapidly (see later in this chapter), but a gradual weaning process is often easier both for the child and for the mother.

How to Wean Young Babies Up to Six or Seven Months
Weaning for young babies is a decision that the mother makes. It is usually easy to carry out. The mother substitutes a bottle-feeding for a nursing each day, and then gradually replaces other nursings until all nursings have been replaced. A mother who plans to wean her young baby to a bottle needs to ensure that her baby will accept a bottle by offering one once or twice per week from early on.

1. The mother begins by *substituting* a bottle, holding and cuddling for one nursing each day. For a baby old enough to have a favorite and less favorite nursing, she should pick a less favorite one to substitute first.

2. She should *watch* to see if there is any reaction in the baby (rash spitting up a lot of milk, bowel problems). She should watch for any emotional reactions (increased thumb sucking, crying, clinging).

She can then substitute at a second feeding each day, after her breasts have adjusted to the lowered demand with less milk. This is usually two to three to five days later. Women may be advised to wait at least a week before adding each new substitution and many women are content with that rate. However, some women are unwilling to accept such a slow pace. If, at the beginning of the weaning process, the baby is nursing eight times/day, and if the mother waits one week between substitutions, weaning will not be completed until approximately two months have gone by. Often when women say, "I have decided to wean," they do not want the weaning process to last two months.

The mother needs to keep watching the baby for any reactions. She will continue to substitute a bottle for an additional daily feeding every several days until no more nursings remain. Weaning ideally is gradual enough to avoid an unhappy frustrated baby or full or tender breasts. Sometimes hand expression is helpful.

It is sometimes better to slow the weaning to a schedule of making a new substitution every five to seven days rather than to persist and have a miserable baby or uncomfortable breasts.

A mother who has almost fully weaned but notices that her baby is having adverse reactions to formula can "unwean." Even if she has only a small amount of milk, she can rebuild her milk supply. It does however require a lot of time with the baby at the breast (see Relactation, Chapter 13). Occasionally, a woman who thought she wanted to wean changes her mind because she misses the nursing. In such cases, women have reversed the weaning process and gone back to full nursing. Most women, however, do complete the weaning process once it is begun; they often report that they miss the nursings but are also glad to have weaned. It is not uncommon for some women, especially those who wean rapidly, to appear to be mildly depressed.

How to Wean an Older Baby—Around Nine Months

At about nine months, many infants seem to "lose interest" in the breast (or bottle). They are beginning to crawl and explore their environment. It is easy to substitute for breastfeedings with a cup or with a bottle (if he is accustomed to it). A mother wishing to wean can usually do so fairly easily.

Some babies in this same age range, however, do not lose interest in nursing; they love to nurse. Some mothers are happy to continue nursing. The problem comes when a baby who shows no inclination toward giving up any nursings is the child of:

1. parents who find nursing older babies or toddlers unappealing and unattractive,
2. a mother who is beginning to feel resentful toward nursing,
3. a mother who is pregnant and who wants to wean.

The mother must decide if she wants to re-evaluate and continue to nurse, or to wean. If she decides to wean, she may need information and support.

Taking advantage of the baby's interest in the rest of the world makes daytime nursings the easiest ones for which to find substitutes. Bedtime nursings are often important to the baby, and it is best to save these for last in weaning. Most babies keep one or two favorite nursings for a longer period and weaning may slow towards the end. Some babies complete the weaning process in a month, some will take many months.

The question of whether to substitute a cup or a bottle will vary with the needs of the child. In any case, a bottle or a cup is a poor substitute unless the mother understands that the baby must have her attention and love along with it. There are pros and cons for both the bottle and the cup. The older baby may still have a strong sucking need and benefit from a bottle. A baby who can just manage a couple of sips from a cup is not ready for only the cup. Weaning directly to a cup does spare the mother the further task of weaning the baby from the bottle. Weaning directly to the cup in the period between 9 and 18 months is well acepted by many babies.

How to Wean a Toddler or Older Child
The nursing toddler is sometimes difficult to wean. Part of his self-image is as a nursing person. Weaning for him ideally is more gradual, sometimes taking many months.

Mothers who are nursing toddlers or older children are in general of two types: those who are convinced of the superiority of baby-led weaning and are content to let the child nurse for as long as he wants; they may belong to a breastfeeding support group, such as La Leche. The second group of mothers nursing children are not completely happy with the situation; they may want information on how to wean their toddler. They do not choose to wait until the child loses interest. They may have enjoyed nursing up to two years but want no part of nursing a three or four year old child. "How to" information on weaning toddlers is not widely distributed. If mother is pregnant, she may want to wean quickly.

The same general rule applies here. It is best for the mother to think not of eliminating nursings, but of substituting for each nursing something that is equally good in the eyes of the baby. Again, the least favorite nursing is most easily eliminated. The problem with toddler weaning, however, is finding equally good substitutes.

Daytime nursings are usually the easiest to find substitutes for, such as a story book and a cuddle, or a walk outside. Many women have found that spring and summer are easier times to wean than in colder times because they can go for outings at times when the child might otherwise ask to nurse, sometimes just from boredom. Other daytime substitutes may be a special snack (hopefully a nutritious one) or joining a play group. Firmly stating that nursing is not to occur outdoors, in stores, etc., also can be used to help decrease the number of nursings.

A child who loves to nurse at bedtime can be told to save up Mommy's milk for that time, as a way of eliminating daytime nursings.

Avoid situations that have meant nursing, such as mother in bed in the morning, watching T.V. after dinner, or sitting for a telephone conversation. Changing daily routines is effective in many cases.

The nursings right before nap time or bed time, as mentioned, are the most difficult ones to find substitutes for. Many mothers have found that the simplest way is for them to be out each evening at bedtime. Some just stay in the house out of sight of the toddler; others go out for an hour. Many toddlers and older children will accept being put to bed by their father or some other adult that they know. If the father reads the child a story and gives the child a good night kiss, the substitution often is a success. Putting the child to bed with a sharp "Now you lie down and go to sleep!" is not a good substitute from any child's point of view.

The older child can be talked to. He can be told that he is getting older and that nursing is for little children and babies. Mothers say, "When you're three (or four) you'll be a big boy and won't nurse any more." Some women have gone away for a few days, and when they returned, have said that their milk was all gone. Some women have put a bad-tasting harmless substance, such as cocktail bitters, on their nipples.

An idea that appeals to one woman seems unnatural or unkind to another. Sometimes mothers say that they want to wean or that they are being pressured to wean but refuse all suggestions on how to change the nursing routines. In this case the mother probably has mixed feelings; she wants to wean, but she also wants to keep on nursing. What they may be saying is that mother-led weaning is not something they want to do; they may need help in dealing with their ambivalent feelings or in realizing that what they say they want is not what they are doing. For women in this ambivalent position, baby- or child-led weaning is most often the best alternative.

Weaning involves an interaction between the mother and child, most especially with children older than 18 months. True baby-led weaning probably does not happen after this age. Children who wean after 18 months are almost always receiving some verbal and/or nonverbal clues that weaning is becoming appropriate. But four year old children are more likely than are two or three year old children to give up nursing entirely on their own. When two, three and four year old children wean, they have usually been encouraged to wean, however gradually and however subtly.

A mother can be advised to watch her child for signs that he is going through a period of expansiveness, when the child enjoys mastering new accomplishments, as a time to initiate weaning. On the other hand, when a child is going through a period of wanting to return to babyhood and acts clingy and babyish, this is often the very time when mothers of nursing children begin to question the nursing. There is usually at least one person—the father or a grandmother, who attributes the babyish behavior to the long-term nursing and recommends weaning. Yet the mother needs to understand that when a child is feeling babyish, this may not be an easy time to encourage him to go on to new things.

Mothers who have nursing children should be reminded that babyish behavior is something all children exhibit; nursing does not cause it. The mother can be reassured to know that her child will pass from the current stage of babyish behavior onto a stage of increased expansiveness.

Rapid Weaning

Sometimes it is not possible for a woman to wean her baby gradually, such as in a situation where the woman is placed on long-term drug therapy, or when the baby dies. Although weaning abruptly or "cold turkey" is not recommended if there is any choice, sometimes a rapid wean is necessary. Consequently the woman needs help in managing the rapid reduction in the demand for milk produced by her breasts. There are some suggestions to make to the mother who must wean rapidly.

Suggested Measures for Women
. . . . Who Must Wean Their Babies Rapidly . . . .

1.   Substitute a bottle for every second feeding.

2.   The next day, the woman can eliminate the remaining feedings one by one. Finally, no nursings remain.

3.   Cut down on her intake of liquids.

4.   Watch the breasts for any sign of breast problems— lumpiness or a hard area. This may indicate a plugged duct or even the beginning of a breast infection. If this occurs, it is best to hand express a little milk, if the woman cannot nurse the baby.

After weaning some women go through a period of depression somewhat similar to postpartum depression, perhaps reflecting similar rapid hormonal changes.

THE NURSING STRIKE (SUDDEN REFUSAL TO NURSE)

A nursing strike occurs when a baby suddenly refuses to nurse whenever he is put to the breast. The baby may arch his back and pull away. Often the mother becomes upset and wonders whether his behavior means that he wants to wean, or has weaned. The difference between a nursing strike and weaning is the *suddenness* In weaning, the baby gradually loses interest in nursing; in a strike, the baby's behavior changes suddenly. One day the baby may nurse eight times or more, and the next day he pulls away and will not nurse at all.

Most babies never go on strike; when a strike occurs, this usually is with babies between the ages of 4 and 13 months.

To the mother, the strike is surprising and very upsetting. She feels rejected and has uncomfortably full breasts. Experience has shown that there generally is one or more reasons for a strike. However, if the cause can be found, which may be difficult, the mother still has the task of coaxing the baby back to nursing (unless she decides to have the strike become a permanent wean).

Some contributing factors that have been identified among babies who have gone on a nursing strike are listed below.

. . . . Factors Associated with Nursing Strikes. . . . .

1.   The baby is teething; his gums throb and the nursing action makes the pain worse.

2.   The baby has a head cold and a stuffy nose. Since he cannot breathe through his nose and must breathe through his mouth, nursing becomes almost impossible.

3.   The baby has an undiagnosed ear infection which is painful, especially when he tries to nurse.

4.   The baby has become accustomed to bottles and has decided that the easier sucking action on a bottle is what he prefers.

5.   The baby had bitten the mother and she reacted (in a very human way) by yelling at him and scaring him.

6.   The baby has been waking up at night. The mother decided to let him "cry it out." The baby reacts to being allowed to scream in place of his usual nursing by refusing to nurse altogether.

7.   There has been some change in the family's life, perhaps a move to a new house or some other new stress. (e.g. A lot of loud quarreling by the parents may frighten a baby into refusing to nurse.)

8.   The mother and baby have been separated. (e.g. The mother of an older baby may have returned after a weekend away, with full breasts, to find the baby refusing to nurse at all.)

A nursing strike may last from two to ten days. Sometimes the baby never goes back to nursing; what started as a nursing strike turns into a permanent wean. Whether or not the baby does resume nursing depends on how the mother handles the situation. In most cases where the mother tries to get the baby back on the breast, the baby does resume nursing. The days during which the baby is refusing to nurse are very upsetting, especially for mothers who had wanted to nurse the baby for more months.

After ruling out and/or treating any medical causes, the mother can be advised to take measures to help end a strike. It is important to note that just relieving initial causes may be and often is insufficient to end a strike.

The following will increase the likelihood of a baby resuming nursing.

. . . . .Suggestions to End a Nursing Strike . . . .

1.   Lots of skin contact between mother and baby.

2.   Large amounts of hugging, cuddling, rocking, and calm talking, without trying to put the baby to the breast. Holding a baby in a way that physically forces him back onto the breast will only make him refuse all the more.

3.   Avoiding all bottles if the baby can take liquids from a cup.

4.   Pumping or hand-expressing milk for comfort is usually necessary. It is not advisable to give mother's milk in a cup or bottle to the baby. He knows where he can get some of that.

5.   If the baby is going to nurse again for the first time, it is probably going to be when he is either sleepy or sleeping. The mother can rock the baby to sleep in a rocking chair, as she is sitting with the baby held across her lap similar to being in a nursing position. The mother should not try to get the baby onto the nipple until he is just drifting off to sleep. This technique is often effective. The comfort of being rocked and held while the baby is sleepy may lead the baby to accept the breast himself.

6.   The baby who nurses at night can be put to sleep in the

mother's bed and attempts made to nurse him once he is soundly asleep.

7. For an older baby, nearer to 12 months in age, the mother can take the striker to where other older babies or toddlers can be seen nursing. Infant peer pressure works sometimes.

The baby will probably resume nursing if mother is patient and persistent. Some strikes have gone on for two weeks. Just as the mother had resigned herself to permanent wean, the baby has resumed nursing. As mentioned above, however, some strikes do become permanent weans.

TANDEM NURSING

Nursing during pregnancy is generally discouraged in the Western world. A woman who continues to nurse throughout a pregnancy and then nurses her newborn and toddler together is said to be "tandem nursing." This is a rare phenomenon in Western countries, but is accepted in some other cultures. Some women nurse the older child throughout the pregnancy, while others wean him during the pregnancy but allow him to resume nursing after the birth of the second child.

There are disadvantages to nursing during pregnancy and to tandem nursing. Once a pregnancy has been diagnosed, weaning may be recommended because of a fear that uterine contractions may possibly cause a miscarriage, or later, premature labor. Further, many pregnant nursing mothers develop very sore nipples, a factor that may cause them to encourage weaning. The milk will decrease in quantity and also change in quality and composition, although the milk will revert to the normal composition after the birth of the second baby and breastfeeding starts again (5).

It is a strain on the mother's body to both nurse and be pregnant. She needs an excellent diet, with large amounts of protein, calcium, etc.

The personal reports of women who have tandem-nursed are mixed, yet all speak of some problems. These tend to be more emotional than physical. Some women have felt resentment toward the older child. Some have felt that the nursing relationship with the older child has interfered with the bonding process with the newborn. The mother may feel resentful toward the older child as he joins in on the nursings.

There also are arguments in favor of tandem nursing. Some women want very much to keep nursing and feel that it would be unfair to the older baby to wean him. The mothers realize that the amount of milk their child is getting during pregnancy is small, but feel that the amount of comfort is enormous. Care must be taken after delivery that the younger baby receives adequate milk. The older baby should receive major nutrition from other sources.

A woman who is pregnant and nursing needs to consider both points of view. Most do wean the older child during pregnancy, perhaps not so much from theoretical concerns, as from sore nipples.

A woman who is having a problem with premature uterine contractions may be advised to wean at once. If this happens, the mother and older baby need to find new ways to replace the feeling of closeness and comfort. The older baby may be only three months old and need to be placed on a formula, or the older baby may be four years old.

When the mother of a previously weaned toddler gives birth again, she may wonder how the older child will react to the sight of the new baby at the breast. Some mothers in this position wonder whether they should allow the older child to try to nurse again. Mothers have been advised to allow the child to nurse because it was believed that he would not remember how to nurse and would soon abandon the attempt (16). Many toddlers do try and give up. But some toddlers latch on expertly and want to nurse along with the baby at every feeding. Many toddlers who have not nursed in many months remember how to nurse or learn how to do so. There are women who wish they had never said, "Sure, go ahead and try." Although some women do not object to starting to nurse the older child again, most women in this position report that they felt negative toward the experience.

ONE-SIDED NURSING

One-sided nursing, or nursing on only one breast, happens for one of two reasons. Either the mother has only one functioning breast, or, more commonly, the baby refuses to nurse from the other breast. Women can nurse after a mastectomy. The analogy of twins helps make believeable that one breast is enough.

When a woman with two breasts nurses on one breast only, the other breast stops producing milk, or "dries up." This phenomenon has been more frequently observed in animals with more teats than young. But it also occurs in at least one human culture where custom and habit dictate that only one side is suckled (7). The breast that is stimulated produces milk in abundance. In this case the woman has a very lopsided appearance. She cannot wear clothing that fits tightly without announcing her situation to the world. Some women have padded the other side for cosmetic reasons. The more the baby nurses, the more obvious is the size difference.

Why does one-sided nursing happen to a woman who has two functioning breasts? Why does a baby refuse one breast? In some cases the mother has a flat or inverted nipple and the baby does not like to nurse on it. The mother can be encouraged to use ice and hand shaping and follow other problem-nipple advice to try to get the baby to nurse on his least favorite side. (See Chapter 8) The mother can be encouraged to try different routines, such as putting the baby on his least favorite side when he is most hungry. Some mothers have used honey on the nipple to encourage the baby to nurse (Since honey can no longer be recommended, sugar water may be suggested instead). Many young babies will nurse on a least favorite side, although they may refuse at times. The mother can use the football hold on the least favorite side so that his same cheek is touching the side he prefers, to try to trick the baby into nursing.

Sometimes there does not seem to be any difference between the two nipples and breasts. It is very rare for a newborn to nurse on one side and refuse the other side when there is no anatomic difference. The mother should keep trying to get the baby to nurse. If the newborn continues to refuse one breast despite all the mother's efforts and there is no abnormality of the shunned nipple, there may possibly be an undiagnosed condition in that breast. (Careful examination of the breast is appropriate, as personal experience has shown a clinical correlation with breast cancer in this situation. The refusal to a newborn to nurse at a flat or inverted nipple, as well as the refusal of an older baby to nurse at one breast are relatively common occurences, and are not suggestive of breast pathology.)

Older babies are much more likely to prefer one breast. There may be a problem with the nipple, or there may be a mole that the baby does not like. In some cases the mother has got into the habit of nursing more on the left side, for example, in order to have her right hand free for other chores. Where there does not seem to be any reason for an older baby to prefer one breast, the theory is that his action is related to being right or left handed.

Summary of Suggestions for Getting Babies
. . . . to Nurse on Least Favorite Side. . . . .

1.   Try nursing him on the less favored side first. Try nursing him when he is sleepy or sleeping.

2.   Try the football hold.

3.   Try nursing in a dark room (for an older baby).

4.   Try switching sides while he's sleeping.

References

General References Used in Preparing the *Ages and Stages section:*

Bowlby, J: *Attachment and Loss.* New York: Basic Books, Inc., 1969.

Bowlby, J. The Nature of the child's tie to his mother, Int. J. Psychoanal. 39:350, 1958.

Brazelton, TB: *Infants and Mothers*. New York: Dell Publishing Co., 1969.

Brazelton, TB: *Toddlers and Parents*. New York: Dell Publishing Co., 1974.

Caplan, F, general editor: *The First Twelve Months of Life*. New York: Grosset & Dunlap, 1973.

Dunn, J: *Distress and Comfort*. Cambridge, Mass.: Harvard Univer. Press, 1977.

Fraiberg, SH: *The Magic Years*. New York: Charles Scribner's Sons, 1959.

Gesell, A: *The First Five Years of Life*. New York: Harper & Brothers Publishers, 1940.

Mussen, PH et al: *Child Development and Personality*. New York: Harper & Row, 1969.

Newton, N: *The Family Book of Child Care*. New York: Harper & Row, 1957.

Piaget, J: *The origins of Intelligence in Children*. New York: International Universities Press, Inc., 1962.

Pryor, K: *Nursing Your Baby*. New York: Pocket Book Division of Simon & Schuster, 1973.

Schaffer, R: *Mothering*. Cambridge, Mass.: Harvard University Press, 1977.

Stone, LJ and Church, J: *Childhood & Adolescence*. New York: Random House, 1968.

Thevenin, T: *The Family Bed*. Minneapolis: Tine Thevenin, P. O. Box 16004, Minneapolis, 1976.

White, B: *First Three Years of Life*. Englewood Cliffs, NJ: Prentice-Hall, Inc., 1975.

Specific References:

1. Fraiberg, S: *The Magic Years*. New York: Charles Scribner's Sons, 1959, pp. 35-36.

2. American Academy of Pediatrics Committee on Nutrition: Flouride Supplementation: Revised Dosage Schedule. Pediatrics 63, 1979.

3. Thevenin, T: *The Family Bed*. Minneapolis: Tine Thevenin, Box 16004, 1976.

4. Jelliffe, DB and Jelliffe, EFP: Biological Night Feeding. J. Trop. Pediatr. 22 (2), 1976.

5. Petros-Barvazian, A. in Changes in the body and its organs during lactation: nutritional implications. CIBA Foundation Symposium 45: 103, 1976.

6. Pryor, K: *Nursing Your Baby*. New York: Pocket Books, 1973.

7. Ing, R et al: (Letter) Unilateral suckling and breast cancer. Lancet 2:655, Sept. 1977.

Chapter 13

Relactation and
Induced Non-Puerperal Lactation

GENERAL DISCUSSION

The term *relactation* refers to the process of restimulating lactation and a milk supply in a woman who no longer is lactating. The term *non-puerperal lactation* refers to inducing lactation in a woman who has not experienced childbirth (1).

Induced lactation and relactation have been reported in primitive cultures, and while relactation is uncommon in Western countries, it is a relatively common occurence in some primitive cultures.

Before discussing the procedures involved in relactation, it may be appropriate to consider the relation of sucking stimulation to milk supply. Induced lactation in a nulliparous woman for an adopted infant is one end of a spectrum; increased milk production during an infant's growth spurt is at the other end. In both cases sucking stimulation by the infant is responsible for inducing milk production. Nursing an adopted infant depends upon providing enough stimulation to create a milk supply where none existed. It can be shown experimentally that nulliparous women who massage or pump their breasts can have a prolactin response similar to that of the nursing, lactating woman (2).

RELACTATION WITH THE MOTHER'S OWN INFANT

Relactation for the woman's own young infant occurs in cases in which the woman either chose not to breastfeed, or weaned prematurely and later wants to put the infant to the breast, usually because of multiple formula intolerance. Since the mother in this case has given birth fairly recently, she will probably be able to rebuild her supply if the infant can be encouraged to keep nursing and if the mother is sufficiently motivated.

A certain percentage of the women who attempt to relactate for their own infants become discouraged and abandon the procedure. This may reflect a basic aversion to breastfeeding in their original choice to bottle feed, in addition to the difficulties in relactation. In considering relactation, it is important to discuss motivation. The woman should be told that relactation requires a great deal of time and effort especially in the beginning. Additional information and first-hand advice and experience are available in *The Tender Gift* (1); *Relactation: A Guide to Breastfeeding the Adopted Baby* (3), and *Induced Lactation: A Guide for Counseling and Management* (4). The relactating woman may, in addition, be referred to a breastfeeding support group. Clearly, a well motivated mother, who understands the process, the difficulties and rewards, can be encouraged to attempt relactation. If the baby is young and willing to suckle, she stands a good chance of success (5).

RELACTATION FOR AN ADOPTED CHILD

If the woman has nursed one or more biological children or is still nursing a toddler, relactation is relatively easy to manage with a young adopted baby. The mother's breasts have undergone the normal physiological changes of lactation, although this advantage may be somewhat lost if many months have passed since the last lactation. Also, such a mother is likely to be well-motivated and knowledgeable about nursing.

INDUCED NON-PUERPERAL LACTATION

Induced non-puerperal lactation is lactation attempted by a nulliparous woman without the benefit of breast development through prior nursing. It has been suggested that the breast must be primed to respond to prolactin (as with a pregnancy that ended in therapeutic or spontaneous abortion), or milk will not be produced (6). Cases of non-puerperal lactation that have been reported and which have received publicity have been those in which the mother has been able to produce milk (7), or what is assumed to be milk.

Biochemical analysis of the breast secretions from women who have induced lactation would be required to determine if these secretions are the same as milk from a normally lactating woman. Phillips, who has studied non-puerperal lactation among the Aborigines of Australia, and other cases of relactation, reports that the first fluid obtained from the breasts after hand expressing may be either a yellowish fluid (resembling colostrum), or it may look like breast milk (8).

The publicity in cases of successful induced lactation is counterbalanced by reports of the women who abandoned the process of inducing lactation as too time-consuming and too frustrating to both mother and child.

Some Arguments Against
. . . . Induced Lactation for Nulliparas . . . .

1.   Induced lactation, especially in a nulliparous woman, is very time-consuming; enormous amounts of stimulation are required to begin the secretion of milk. The time might be better spent in other ways of interacting within the family. The rewards of inducing lactation may or may not be exceeded by the difficulties.

2.   Many of those nulliparous women who attempt to relactate abandon the procedure; often they do it with some sense of failure. To the infertile woman, this may seem one more example of her inability in physical functioning as a woman.

3.   Adoptive parents are sometimes advised that they will develop a good parent-child relationship most readily by acknowledging they have adopted rather than by trying to deny this circumstance (9).

MANAGEMENT OF RELACTATION AND INDUCED LACTATION

Management involves the same procedures, whether the woman is relactating or inducing lactation for the first time. Nursing an adopted baby is considered to be easier for women who have previously nursed one or more biological children in terms of the number of ounces produced, but this may not always be so (3,4). Relactation is a time-consuming process requiring patience and true commitment. Both women who have nursed previously and those who have not nursed should be encouraged to think in terms of their relationship with the adopted child. The emphasis should not be on the number of ounces of milk produced. The child may need to receive all or nearly all of his nourishment from supplementary sources and yet still can benefit psychologically from nursing at the breast.

However, women who understand that the nursing relationship with an adopted child is more important than the number of ounces produced may still want to know what the chances are that they will be able to build up an adequate milk supply. Creating or recreating a milk supply depends upon both the mother and the baby. It is essential that the baby cooperate by sucking vigorously for long periods of time. The ideal baby for a relactation would be a healthy newborn with a strong sucking need. A baby older than a few weeks is unlikely to provide the sucking stimulation required; he also would be accustomed to bottle feeding and is unlikely to cooperate. In many cases where relactation or induced lactation has been abandoned, the cause was the infant's refusal to cooperate by suckling at empty breasts.

A woman who would like to induce lactation for an adopted baby may prepare her breasts before the infant arrives, more effectively if she knows approximately when she will receive the adopted baby. Breast massage, hand expression, and the use of a breast pump have been suggested. Chloropromazine may aid in developing the milk supply by inhibiting PIF and causing prolactin levels to rise (10,11). The effect of drugs may also be a psychological one. Estrogens, in the form of oral contraceptives in a limited dosage, have been prescribed for nulliparous women before the baby arrives in an attempt to prepare the breasts (3).

Whether the mother is attempting to relactate or to induce lactation, the same principles apply. The baby is put to the breast as often as he will cooperate and nurse. This may be every two hours. To entice the infant to nurse at an empty breast, sugar water can be used on the nipple. Or the woman may be advised to use an eye dropper to squirt milk into the corner of the baby's mouth. The Lact-Aid (described in Chapter 14) eliminates the need for sugar water or eye droppers.

A baby who prefers the bottle may be more cooperative in suckling at the breast when he is sleepy or even sleeping. Some babies who are accustomed to bottles only will not cooperate in nursing, with or without the Lact-Aid.

Ideally, the mother wears the Lact-Aid at each feeding; the stimulation received causes a gradual increase in her milk supply. Ideally, smaller and smaller amounts of the supplementary formula are needed. It is important to counsel the woman against trying too hard to eliminate the supplement, or dilute the formula. "Throwing away the bottles" or cutting back on the amount of supplement quickly may be effective in an occasional case of relactation, but it can result in undernutrition and or dehydration. Diluting the supplement may make the infant gradually weaker and placid, rather than more eager at the breast (4).

The infant must be checked frequently. The characteristics of the infant's stools, whether of the breastfed or bottle-fed type, may help in assessing whether the mother is producing appreciable amounts of milk.

In some cases of relactation, the multiparous woman has been able to rebuild her milk supply to the point where the infant is taking only a small amount of supplement per day and is making good weight gains. A mother whose baby is taking the equivalent of one bottle per day may hesitate to give up the last supplement. She should realize that if she is able to satisfy the infant 90%, she will be able to satisfy him 100%. She may simply lack the confidence to give up the final bottle.

The woman who can meet only 50% of the baby's needs after several weeks of relactation may need to accept the continued need to give supplemental foods, usually formula.

WET NURSING AS AN AID TO RELACTATION
AND INDUCED LACTATION

Wet nursing, or the nursing of a baby by a woman other than the mother, has been used as a way to relactate or induce lactation. Wet nursing has been practiced for as long as recorded history. Before the bottle became available in the twentieth century a wet nurse was the only safe alternative when a natural mother could not nurse her baby.

Wet nursing as an aid to relactation or induced lactation has been effective. A woman who has little or no milk swaps babies with a woman who has an adequate milk supply. The baby who is used to nursing at his mother's full breasts cooperates (hopefully) by sucking at the empty breasts of the other woman. He is essentially using her as a pacifier and gives her valuable breast stimulation. Meanwhile, the woman with milk nurses the other baby and shows him that milk does come from breasts, instead of just bottles. The nursing mother gains the satisfaction of giving herself and her milk to someone who needs it. In cases of severe allergy to formulas, the mother is giving the baby a food he can thrive on. The mother wishing to induce milk production gains breast stimulation.

It seems at first that wet nursing is so effective in cases of relactating that it ought to return to popularity. Yet the practice is rarely recommended. There are arguments against wet nursing:

. . . . Arguments Against Wet Nursing. . . . .

1. The mothers and babies are being exposed to different bacterial environments. Transmission of certain viruses in breast milk has been documented.

2. Swapping nursing babies between different mothers can confuse the babies. One case involved baby swapping and donations of breast milk from 10 different mothers (12).

3. There are other options available today: the Lact-Aid (to encourage sucking stimulation) — and breast milk from a milk bank (in cases where a baby cannot tolerate any formula) can be made available.

References

1. Raphael, D: *The Tender Gift: Breastfeeding.* Englewood Cliffs, New Jersey: Prentice Hall, 1973.

2. Noel, GL et al: Prolactin release during nursing and breast stimulation in postpartum and nonpostpartum subjects, J. Clin. Endocrinol. Metab. 38:413, 1974.

3. Hormann, E: *Relactation: A Guide to Breastfeeding the Adopted Baby.* Elizabeth Hormann, 1971.

4. Avery, JL: *Induced Lactation: A Guide for Counseling and Management.* Denver: J.J. Avery, Inc. 1973.

5.   Herman, E: Relactation: How To Do It, The Lactation Review I (1), 1976.

6.   Tyson, JE in Hormonal Control of Lactation, CIBA Foundation Symposium 45:49, 1976.

7.   Krensky, L: *Adopted Baby*. Philadelphia: CEA of Greater Philadelphia, 1969.

8.   Phillips, V: *Successful Breast Feeding*. Victoria, Australia: Nursing Mothers' Association of Australia, 1976.

9.   Carey, WB: A Point of View, in Three Commentaries Concerning Breast-Feeding Adopted Infants. Conshohocken: CEA of Greater Philadelphia.

10. Brown, RE: Breast feeding in modern times, Am. J. Clin. Nutr. 26:556, 1973.

11. Waletzky, LR: Relactation, Amer. Family Physician 14: (2), 1976.

12. Robinson, TM: I Nursed Our Adopted Son. Philadelphia: CEA of Greater Philadelphia.

Chapter 14

Devices and Miscellaneous Topics

With the possible exception of bottles and pacifiers, most or all of the devices discussed in this chapter are not needed by the majority of breast-feeding women. The material is here for reference and for use in managing occasional problems. The following topics are covered:

Bottles and pacifiers
Breast shields and nipple shields
The milk cup
Breast pumps
Breast massage and the hand expression of breast milk
Storing breast milk
Donor milk
Milk banks
Bra pads
Lact-aid

A list of products, and their manufacturers and addresses, is found in Appendix B.

BOTTLES

Many breastfeeding women also use bottles regularly for their babies, but others nurse for months without using a single bottle. Some women feel comfortable providing a bottle of hand-expressed breast milk, but guilty leaving formula for the sitter. It often is convenient, however, to leave ready-to-use bottles of formula.

There are advantages in using bottles regularly for the breastfed baby, as well as disadvantages. With the exception of specific medical indications for additional nutrients or fluids, the use of supplemental bottles is a decision appropriately made by informed parents. It is not really a medical decision.

Arguments against Supplemental Bottles

There are arguments against the use of regular bottles, especially in the puerperium—arguments that are infrequently told to mothers. Too often a new mother has lacked confidence in the adequacy of her milk supply and has given the infant a bottle to "fill him up" (1,2). Dr. Niles Newton has described the route by which one bottle usually leads to another. There is some evidence that many babies who receive a bottle twice/week early on will be totally bottle fed by three or four months of age. Psychologically, the feeling of "You belong to me and I belong to you and there are no substitutes" disappears (1).

There is an additional reason for avoiding bottles in the puerperium. Two different types of mouth actions are required in suckling at the breast and sucking on a rubber nipple (3). (See Fig. 14-1) Requiring the infant to learn two different ways of sucking confuses some infants. The baby who is fed with bottles develops a measurably weaker sucking reflex by four days of age, so that he sucks less vigorously at the breast (4).

A mother whose nipples are flat or inverted is particularly at a disadvantage when her infant is alternately given the supernormal stimulus of the rubber nipple and then her own poorly protractile nipple. Sucking on a bottle nipple is easier for any infant and may make the infant unwilling to make the effort to nurse at the mother's breast (5). An effective way to reduce the incidence of infants who "won't nurse" or "refuse the breast" is to avoid the routine use of bottles in the first week.

Arguments for Supplemental Bottles

Women often are told that every breastfed baby should become accustomed to taking a bottle. If the mother of a completely breastfed baby should be unable to return home for a feeding, or if she should be hospitalized, or if she should die, the baby would be left without his only source of nourishment. Babies who are not accustomed to regular bottles have often been observed to refuse the bottle.

Many women do want to be able to go out occasionally, or want to be able to have someone else give occasional feedings and prefer to accustom their babies to accept a bottle. A further argument in favor of the use of regular bottles is that this allows the baby's father the opportunity to feed the baby.

Good general advice about bottles is that bottles should be offered from a position of strength, not weakness. An example of a position of strength:

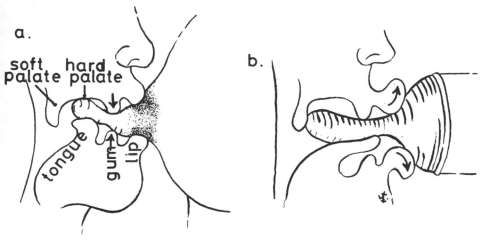

a.

soft hard
palate palate

tongue gum lip

b.

Figure 14-1. Diagrams of the sucking mechanism at the breast. (a) The tongue thrusts forward to grasp the nipple and areola. The nipple is brought against the hard palate as the tongue pulls backward, bringing the areola into the mouth. Negative pressure is created by the action of the tongue and cheeks against the nipple, and the result is s true sucking action. The gums compress the areola, squeezing milk into the back of the throat. Milk flows against the hard palate from the high pressure system of the breast to the area of negative pressure at the back of the throat. (b) In contrast, the large rubber nipple of a bottle strikes the soft palate (causing gagging) and interferes with the action of the tongue. The tongue moves forward against the gum to control the overflow of milk into the esophagus. The lips are flanged into an "O" shape; compression does not occur, because the cheek muscles are relaxed. (after Applebaum)

the mother is confident that she has enough milk; she wants to go out for a few hours and will be away from the baby. The bottle is appropriate. An example of a position of weakness: the mother either does not have, or fears she docs not have enough milk; she turns to a bottle in the hope of filling up a hungry baby. This mother needs advice on milk supply, not advice on bottle preparation. A woman who has a low milk supply, or who has doubts about her milk supply, needs to be told that bottles will never build up a milk supply. Many women need to be reassured that the later afternoon or early evening feeding is smaller for other women too, and that this is normal. Women need to be reassured that the baby can receive less milk at some feedings than at others. Parents need to understand that some infants will accept bottles even when they are not hungry because of their strong sucking need, just as they will take a pacifier or thumb: women who try to give a bottle after a nursing are discouraged when the baby accepts it!

Women who decide that they want to accustom their babies to accepting the bottle ought not to begin giving the bottles until the end of the second week, after the infant has learned to suckle. Then a bottle can be offered approximately twice a week, or as often as once a day without interfering with the mother's milk supply. The crucial point is that the mother understand what she is doing, that she understand the supply and demand concept—how one bottle can possibly lead to another. She can then make rational decisions about what her style of nursing will be.

If she notices that her baby is beginning to prefer the bottle (not uncommon around 4 months, and not uncommon for working mothers), or if she notices that her milk supply is dwindling, then she can decide how to manage the situation. She can either increase the number of nursings, if she wants the breastfeeding experience to continue, or she can continue with regular bottles, which is a gradual weaning process.

PACIFIERS

Pacifiers (called comforters in the United Kingdom) can be useful during lactation, but mothers who find them unattractive can meet all of the sucking needs of their infants with the breast.

The circumstances of the nursing mother sometimes suggest the possible use of a pacifier. A new mother may need to use a pacifier to satisfy her baby's sucking need when her nipples are too sore to continue nursing after five or ten minutes of nursing. A nursing mother may offer a pacifier when she is in a situation where she would be embarrassed to nurse, although many women learn to nurse modestly in various public places. A nursing mother may need to go out to do a quick errand while someone else stalls off the baby for a few minutes. Women who choose not to continue nursing after 10 or 20 or 30 minutes because of other responsibilities may use pacifiers.

The circumstances of the nursing baby may also indicate the possible use of a pacifier. A pacifier is indicated for the infant who has ingested so much breast milk that he is spitting up but still wants to suck. An infant who is overweight may need less milk but more sucking. In both of these cases the pacifier can be useful. An alternative, in both cases, would be to allow the infant to suck for a longer period of time, but only at one breast per nursing.

The combination of the strong early sucking need and the widespread occurence of sore nipples makes the puerperium the appropriate time for introducing the pacifier, for those women who decide that they would like to do so.

One brand of pacifier, the Nuk Exercisor, is said to have the same shape as a mother's nipple inside the infant's mouth during breastfeeding and may be better accepted by a nursing infant than a traditionally shaped pacifier. Any pacifier will be better accepted if the infant is held while it is being offered. (A string to keep the pacifier around the baby's neck must never be used as this can cause choking and death. Only pacifiers that are well made and sturdy should be used.)

The risk in the use of pacifiers for nursing infants is inadequate stimulation of mother's milk supply. Inadvertently, the mother may use the pacifier too much and the milk supply may dwindle through lack of sucking stimulation. Infants who are given pacifiers to fulfill their sucking needs sometimes are not allowed to suckle long enough at the breast to maintain the milk supply and to cause the supply to increase with the baby's increasing appetite (6).

Women may inadvertently fail to provide enough stimulation to their breasts (7) and may resort to cereal or bottles to fill up the baby.

In a typical situation where the pacifier is causing a problem, the baby is nursing just long enough to get the milk that comes quickly and easily as the milk lets-down at the beginning of each nursing. The mother gets into the habit of slipping in the pacifier—"putting in the plug"—so that the baby becomes less and less willing to suck on a relatively empty breast and thinks of the breast as a source of food only, not as a source of comfort or sucking satisfaction. The mother often thinks of the breast in the same limited way. The mother does not understand that the type of sucking that babies usually do near the end of a feeding—when they seem to be sleepy, when their jaws are barely moving and alternate sucking and resting—is important to maintaining the milk supply.

Wolfe described two different types of sucking patterns of infant mammals; these are the nutritive mode, when the milk is flowing, and the non-nutritive mode, when little or no milk is flowing (8).

Most breastfeeding mothers using the pacifier will do so appropriately. But problems with milk supply are more likely to happen with infants who spend a great deal of time sucking on a pacifier (6).

BREAST SHIELDS AND NIPPLE SHIELDS

The terms "breast shield" and "nipple shield" often are confused. In a telephone conversation with a woman with a problem with a shield, the important question to ask is "What does it look like?" What you picture as a breast shield or a nipple shield may not be what the woman is using.

The milk cup is called a breast shield by some. It is made of clear, hard plastic. It is described and illustrated in Chapter 5 (see Fig. 5-3). The term "milk cup" will be used in this handbook for this clear, hard plastic device, in order to differentiate it from other devices. The funnel-shaped part of a breast pump that is placed at the breast is also called a breast shield by some manufacturers. In this handbook, the term "flange" will be used for the funnel-shaped part of a breast pump (see Fig. 14-6).

For clarity, the term "breast shield" will be used *only* for the all-rubber, floppy shield. These all-rubber devices are called breast shields by their manufacturers and commonly are found in pharmacies (see Fig. 14-2).

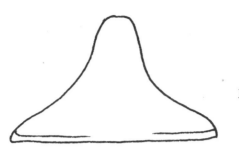

Figure 14-2. A breast shield.

The term "nipple shield" will be used for the combination rubber and plastic shield also found in pharmacies (see Fig. 14-3).

Both breast shields and nipple shields can be useful if used correctly, but there is a great deal of confusion about why and how to use any kind of shield. The correct indication for the use of a nipple or breast shield is to draw out a flat, inverted, or semi-inverted nipple. The nipple shield works better than the breast shield for this purpose. The woman wets the shield for better contact with her breast and places the shield directly over the problem nipple. The baby is then able to grasp hold of the shield, whereas he may not have been able to grasp the woman's own nipple. The baby's sucking draws the woman's nipple outward into the shield. Then, once the nipple is drawn out, the shield is quickly removed and the baby put back onto the woman's formed nipple (9). Using the correct procedure is vital but the box in which the shield is packaged usually gives no instructions and does not mention the need to remove the shield promptly.

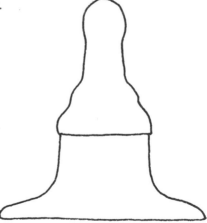

Figure 14-3. A nipple shield.

Reasons for Not Letting a Baby
. . . . Keep Nursing Through a Shield . . . .

1. The shield interferes with proper stimulation and so interferes with conditioning or triggering of the let-down reflex.

2.   A baby usually obtains very little milk for many minutes of sucking through a shield.

3.   The breast is not well-emptied and so engorgement is more likely to develop. Engorgement makes any nipple seem flatter and thus more difficult for the baby to grasp.

4.   Infants quickly become accustomed to the size and shape of the shield, the feel of the rubber. A shield is so easy to grasp hold of that infants sometimes refuse to cooperate in drawing out the woman's own nipple. A woman with a single flat or an inverted nipple or with problems with both nipples especially needs a cooperative baby.

Removing the shield as soon as the nipple is drawn out will prevent the above problems.

Sometimes a baby becomes "hooked" on a breast shield. To undo this problem (which leads to a dwindling milk supply), the mother can coax the baby to nurse without it, or she can use a pair of small scissors to cut away part of the rubber tip of the shield. She should be advised to begin at the center of the nipple part. The baby nurses with the center tip cut out. Before each subsequent feeding, a little more of the rubber is cut away, always from the center outward. Thus, increasing amounts of the woman's own nipple are exposed. Finally there is little left to the rubber of the shield except for the outer rim.

The technique of weaning from the shield by cutting it away is effective, but weaning from the shield can be frustrating because the baby acts fussy and cries. The problem is best avoided by never allowing women to keep nursing through any shield.

Should a shield (and advice on its use) be offered to all women with problem nipples? Probably not. There are better methods to try first. They are better because they do not involve anything coming between the mother and the baby and because they do not involve any danger of the baby refusing to nurse without the shield.

Better Alternatives to the Breast Shield
. . . . .and Nipple Shield . . . .

1.   Correct nipple preparation during pregnancy is most effective. If a woman delivers without having been told about and/or without having done any nipple preparation to draw her retracted nipples out during pregnancy, she should be advised to use the Hoffman technique and to wear a milk cup between and just before feedings.

2.   Advise the woman to use cold, such as crushed ice in a clean cloth, or just a cold cloth, to help her nipples become erect or come out as much as possible prior to nursings.

3.   Along with the cold, have the woman hand shape her nipple with her fingers before putting it into the baby's mouth. She can also use her two fingers to compress the area behind the nipple, the "scissor hold," to try to get the nipple well back into the baby's mouth.

4.   Help the woman avoid engorgement, which makes any nipple more difficult to grasp. The woman can wear a milk cup between nursings (and especially just before a nursing) to depress the area around the nipple and encourage the nipple to extend outward, if she is becoming engorged.

A shield is not an appropriate suggestion for sore nipples. The idea of using a shield to "protect" the nipples from irritation in case of sore nipples is based on good intentions but fallacious reasoning. The shield itself can be irritating where the rubber is in contact with the skin. Often the shield shifts slightly as the baby nurses and this rubbing can be uncomfortable. Also, 20 minutes of nursing through a shield may yield no more milk than 5 minutes without it. So, a shield, if overused, can increase or cause problems instead of curing them. Some women, however, may hesitate to nurse at all if they have sore nipples. They may be better off if they agree to nurse with a shield than not to nurse at all. However, there are other ways to prevent, as well as cure, soreness (see Chapter 8).

Because shields have gained a reputation for causing more problems than they cure, some hospitals no longer stock shields at all for the maternity unit. This arrangement has the advantage that inexperience personnel can not hand out shields for inappropriate reasons. Instead, the hospitals stock milk cups for problem nipples that need to be encouraged to stand out.

MILK CUP (ALSO SOMETIMES CALLED A BREAST SHIELD)

The milk cup is similar to the older Woolwich breast shield. It is worn during pregnancy or between nursings (see Fig. 5-3). As discussed in the previous section, it is confusing to call three diferent types of devices "shields," so the term "milk cup," which is already in use by some manufacturers, seems preferable for the clear, hard plastic device.

Although breast shields and nipple shields are worn over the mother's own nipple at the beginning of a nursing, the milk cup is never worn during a nursing. It is worn in the last months of pregnancy, or in the puerperium, by a woman with one or two non-protractile nipples to encourage the nipple(s) to stand out. The steady gentle pressure of the inside rim of the cup forces the nipple to extend forward.

The milk cup also can be used for an entirely different use, that is, to collect milk that leaks from the second breast as the mother nurses. The collection of milk was the original use of such devices in the Victorian era (10). The milk cup from CEA of Greater Philadelphia has instructions on this additional use. Some devices, identical to the milk cup, however, are not packaged with such instructions but can be used for this purpose also. devices, but in the opinions of those who have written the instructions. The original use of such devices during the Victorian era was to collect milk that leaked from the breasts between feedings (10).

If the woman plans to save the milk that leaks from the second breast, the cup must be sterilized before it is inserted into the bra. Milk collected in a non-sterile cup *must* be discarded. The cup should be positioned so that the little air hole is at the top. With proper attention to sterilizing, the milk may be saved. Immediately after a nursing, the leaked milk is poured into a sterile container and chilled. When it is cold, it can be added as a new layer to any already frozen milk in the freezer. Milk that is collected in this way is subject to no more handling than is milk that a mother hand-expresses and freezes in preparing a bottle. Obviously milk that has been allowed to sit at body temperature must be discarded.

A woman using a breast pump on one breast could insert a sterilized milk cup into the bra on the "other" side to collect leaking milk, in addition to the pumped milk (11).

Women who have leaking problems between feedings have sometimes worn the cups all the time to keep the clothing dry. This is a poor idea. The pressure on the skin around the nipple (the same pressure that forces an inverted nipple outward) can actually encourage more leaking by the constant pressure on the area over the lacteal sinuses. The only women who should wear the cups regularly between feedings are those whose nipples continue to invert or lack protractility postpartum.

Commercial advertisements for milk cups advise unsuspecting mothers to use the devices for inappropriate uses, such as for curing sore nipples (which they do not do), and may suggest continual use. Also, commercially advertised ones cost several times as much as those sold by breastfeeding support groups.

BREAST PUMPS
Supporting the Mother

There are two groups of reasons for women expressing breast milk: *baby reasons*, such as prematurity or a cleft palate, and *mother reasons*, such as the mother's need to take contraindicated medication temporarily, her separation from the child, or her wish to donate milk to a milk bank.

If the various methods of removing milk from the breasts were to be compared, only nursing by a baby would be considered to be excellent. No pump is as gentle or effective as a baby, largely because it is very difficult for women to let-down to a pump. Further, it is better for the milk to go directly to the baby rather than being collected and transferred. It is a mistake to substitute a breast pump for a baby unless there is a problem with the baby which makes suckling impossible (cleft palate, prematurity). Sore nipples and mastitis are not indications for using a pump.

Breast pumping, and to a certain extent, breastfeeding itself, are unfamiliar techniques. The woman who is about to express her milk is often worried both about her infant and the pump. She needs information and a support person who is familiar with the breast pump and breast pumping. Unfortunately, knowing how to nurse does not automatically lead anyone to an understanding of how to pump; making the assumption that the pumping experience is like the nursing experience can lead to problems. Medical and lay counselors might benefit from involvement in a workshop, in order to clearly differentiate advice that is appropriate for mothers of healthy term infants from advice that is appropriate for mothers of sick or premature infants.

The significant fact about breast pumps that needs to be stressed is that the pump is not a baby. The pumping experience is unlike the nursing experience in the following significant ways:

. . . .Ways in Which Pumping Differs from Breastfeeding . . . .

1.   Because the pump does not demand attention, there is a tendency for the woman to leave it unused, sitting in the closet, especially after many days or weeks of pumping. Thus, the woman should be advised to put herself on a schedule of every 2-3 hours in the daytime, if she wants to collect milk for the infant. The woman should not, however, set her alarm to get up at night to pump. The analogy to nursing on demand cannot be carried over to the pumping experience!

2.   A significant difference between the pumping and nursing experiences is the difficulty the pumping mother has in conditioning her let-down reflex to an unattractive mechanical device, instead of to a cuddly baby. With pumping it is necessary to use specific compensation measures to aid in conditioning the let-down reflex.

The support person(s) can be most helpful to the mother in helping her to find ways to condition the let-down reflex to the pump:

(a) The pump should be set up where the mother does not feel embarrassed by onlookers, both in the hospital and home settings. The location of the pump can either help the woman to feel more comfortable, or it can prevent her from doing so.

(b) The woman can be advised to use relaxation breathing, or at least to take a few deep breaths.

(c) The woman should be taught to do breast massage before each pumping episode; breast massage also is helpful during a pumping session. Massaging around each breast several times is an effective aid to conditioning the let-down reflex.

(d) Synthetic oxytocin (Syntocinon) can be effective in triggering the let-down reflex (12). This may be administered as one or two sprays from a nasal spray.

In order to imitate the pattern found in normal nursing, Syntocinon can be used more than once during a pumping session.

3. Another major difference between the nursing and pumping experiences is in the reasonable expectation about the number of ounces of milk obtained. Each woman needs to be advised that she will not be able to express as much milk with a breast pump as an infant would be able to suckle. One quarter ounce of colostrum may be a reasonable expectation for a first attempt at pumping. The woman can be advised to use breast massage and to continue pumping but, if after a few minutes no more colostrum or milk can be obtained, the woman should not force herself to continue and so to become discouraged. Pumping for 1 minute after the milk has slowed is long enough.

4. Another major point of difference involves the difference in instructions to be given to nursing and to pumping mothers. With nursing, the mother can be told to nurse on demand, approximately every 2-2½ hours with a newborn. She could nurse with her eyes closed. She can relax at feedings, watch television, and so forth. This is not so with pumping. The woman attaches the pump to one breast; how long she leaves the pump flange there depends on what is happening. The woman has to watch to see whether milk is spraying out. If so, she should leave the flange in place. But if no drops are coming out, the woman should switch to the other breast. If milk can be *seen* to come from the other breast, the woman should quickly switch to that breast so as not to lose that milk. Each mother should be told that the point of pumping is to collect whatever milk there is. This seems to be obvious, but may not be recognized by a distraught mother.

5.   Another major difference between nursing and pumping is the pattern of the mother's milk supply, when the pumping goes on for several weeks, as is common in the case of pumping for a premature infant. In nursing, a woman's milk supply would be fairly easy to predict. Her milk is said to "come in;" then it adjusts to the amount her baby needs and remains at that level, with gradual increases as the baby stimulates increased production.

This is not the case with a woman who is pumping over a period of weeks. Her milk supply may be expected to come in slightly later and the milk supply may not remain at the appropriate high level. In many cases of prolonged pumping, the woman's supply dwindles.

The pump cannot fully duplicate a baby in maintaining a supply, even if the pumping is done on a regular schedule. Emotional factors are involved. In the case of a mother pumping for a premature infant, for example, the supply often follows the baby's prognosis (13). If the mother is told that her baby is not doing well, the mother's emotional reaction may lead to a reduction in the supply. When a mother is told that her infant is doing so well that he can come home in a few days, or that the mother may come into the nursery to nurse him, the mother's emotions often lead to an increase in the supply.

Some of the factors affecting the milk supply of the pumping mother, such as the infant's prognosis, are not easy to control. The one factor that can be controlled effectively is the quality of the support and information that the woman receives from the support person(s) on an on-going basis. With ideal support and information, the milk supply need not dwindle so drastically.

6.   Another difference between the nursing experience and the pumping experience directly involves the support person. With nursing, the mother generally needs less information and support after the first week than she has needed in the first day or two. With pumping, the mother often needs *more* support as the days go by and discouragement becomes likely.

Increased pumping may help a woman to increase her milk supply. The most practical application of this advice comes shortly before an infant is due to be discharged from the hospital. The mother should be urged to step up her pumping schedule and pump one or more times at night in order to stimulate increased milk production.

7.   With a mother who is nursing, the need for the mother's sleep pattern to be disturbed by night feedings should be expected to decrease gradually as the infant grows. With the long-term pumping experience, there may be an increasing need for the mother to get up at night in order to maintain milk production. (The growing infant is able to maintain and even to increase milk supply with fewer nursings.)

Pumping Equipment

All breast pumps have a funnel-shaped flange (also called a "shield") that comes in contact with the mother's nipple. The milk flows along the flange as it comes from the breast. The flange and the collecting jar come in contact with the milk. There is a question of whether glass or plastic is preferable for the parts that come in contact with the milk. Although both of these can be autoclaved, some people support glass, and some support high quality plastic. There is a major objection to each of the two materials. With regard to glass, it is argued that the macrophages in breast milk cling to the walls of the glass and therefore are not available to the infant (14); this is particularly unfortunate for the premature infant for whom breast milk is often collected. The disadvantages of plastic are that it can be scratched and that chemicals of the plastic may also leach into the milk.

The following sections describe the commonly used breast pumps, although there are others.

Electric Pumps

Electric pumps are often considered to be the most efficient; however, they are expensive. Many hospitals have an electric pump for use by maternity patients. Medical supply houses rent them. Childbirth and breastfeeding support groups can often supply information on obtaining or renting a pump.

The pump that is the Rolls Royce of electric pumps is the Egnell—expensive, classy-looking and quiet (see Fig. 14-4). It is manufactured in Europe and is available to buy or rent in the United States and in some European countries. Egnell has a plan for using hospitals, drug stores or breastfeeding groups as rental agents. The pumps are usually equipped with all-plastic parts, although glass parts may be ordered from Egnell. Each mother who rents an Egnell pump receives her own kit of new accessories. The weekly cost of renting an Egnell is higher than most other pumps but may be covered by a few insurance plans, or by public assistance-type payments.

There are other brands of breast pumps available through medical supply houses. Some electric breast pumps are converted lung aspirators.

Electric pumps require a three-hole outlet. An adaptor with a grounding

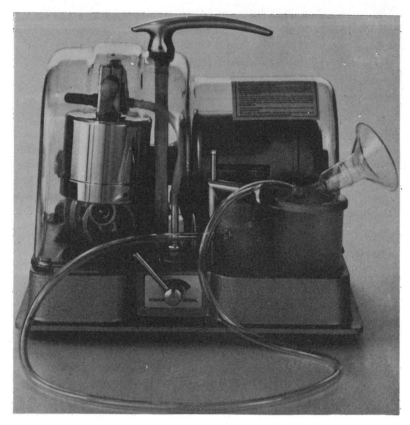

Figure 14-4. The Egnell pump.
(Courtesy Egnell, Inc.)

wire may be used *only* if the outlet is properly grounded for this purpose.

Water-Powered Pumps

There are some small breast pumps available which use water instead of elec-
tricity as the source of power (see Fig. 14-5). The pump attaches to a faucet,
similar to the way an electric portable dishwasher attaches. The faster the
water flows, the stronger the suction.

The Loyd-B Pump

The Loyd-B is a small and inexpensive pump that comes with instructions
(see Fig. 14-6). The parts are glass. The Loyd-B can be purchased, or a
hospital or other agency can act as a rental depot. The main advantages are
the small size, low price, and effective pumping action, which can be regu-
lated from gentle to stronger. It also needs no outside power supply, and is
the only major pump which can be used inside an oxygen tent, because it is
not electric. The Loyd-B is popular with working mothers.

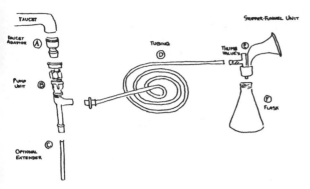

Figure 14-5. A water pump.

The handle of the Loyd-B can be shifted around to a comfortable position. The woman squeezes the trigger handle three to four times to begin the pumping action. After the desired amount of vacuum is obtained, the woman need not continue squeezing the trigger. To release the suction, the woman pulls the small black lever—the vacuum release trigger—toward her. Women with small hands may have difficulty in reaching the release level while holding the Loyd-B pump.

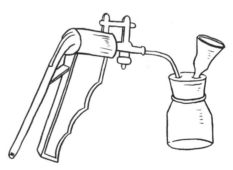

Figure 14-6. The Loyd B pump.

Instruction in the Use of a Breast Pump
Specific instructions vary slightly with different pumps, but pumps have more in common than they may appear to have at first, because they vary so in appearance. All pumps have the same basic features:

. . . . Common Features of Breast Pumps . . . .

1.   A means to create suction and a means to regulate the strength of the suction.

2.   An area for collecting the milk.

3.   A flange that is applied to the breast.

4.   Parts that require sterilization.

All of the above pumps require the same general advice for the woman using them. Unless she is using a hand-pump (covered in the next section), a woman who is about to use any pump should be instructed to do the following:

. . . . Instructions in the Use of a Breast Pump . . . .

1.   Wash your hands. Have all equipment that will come in contact with the milk sterilized according to desired procedure.

2.   Use breast massage (see later this chapter) before beginning to pump. Massage is also very helpful when repeated during a pumping session.

3.   Wet the contact area between the nipple and the flange with sterile water or allow the first drops of milk to flow back along the nipple. This will allow the nipple to slide freely and prevent rubbing. The sliding is important in triggering the let-down.

4.   Do *not* try to center the nipple in the middle of the flange, but let it slide along the inside of the top part of the flange.

5.   Hold the flange just tightly enough to close out the air, but do not press inward so tightly as to dig into the skin. Many women tend to press the lower part of the flange more and more tightly into the skin as the pumping session continues. This would prevent the milk in the lower half of the breast from flowing.
     Each woman needs to be shown how to hold the flange to her breast, tightly enough for a good seal, but not so tightly that she digs the flange into her breast and impedes the flow of the milk. This is a common mistake made by nervous mothers.

6.   Do not fill any collecting jar above the line indicated. The additional milk would then be wasted.

The Hand Pump

The inexpensive hand pump is available at most pharmacies (see Fig. 14-7). It has been nicknamed the "bicycle horn." Many women like the pump for occasional use, but many others find that using it produces an uncomfortable pinching sensation (5). Some women like to use the hand pump while

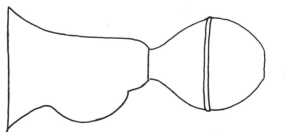

Figure 14-7. A hand pump.

nursing on one side and pumping on the other. They use the milk for occasional bottles to get time away from the baby. A woman who needs to collect milk for a premature infant needs a better pump than a hand pump, as the woman's hand becomes tired quickly.

A further disadvantage is the possibility of bacterial contamination; cleaning the inside of the rubber bulb into which milk often flows inadvertently is not easy. In a study of the bacterial count of banked human milk, it was found that milk obtained with a rubber-bulb breast pump had a significantly greater degree of bacterial contamination than milk collected by hand expression. In the milk obtained by hand expression, the mean colony count was 2,500 colonies/ml. In the milk collected with the pump, the mean colony count was 135,000 colonies/ml. Cultures from sterile washes of "clean" rubber suction bulbs of the hand pumps had counts greater than 1,000,000 colonies/ml (15).

. . . . Instructions in the Use of a Hand Pump. . . . .

1. Wash the hands. Sterilize the pump and any container used for collecting and storing the milk.

2. Massage the breast. Some women like to use hand-expression in addition to breast massage in order to get the flow started before putting the hand pump to the breast.

3. Hold the pump by the bulb end with the collecting area held down. The pump should be held such that the nipple is sliding along the inside of the top of the flange, for contact, to trigger the let-down. The spout can be moistened with sterile water, or the first few drops of milk can be allowed to wet the inside of the flange.

4. Squeeze the bulb gently—no more than half way—and place the pump over the nipple.

5. Gently release the squeeze on the bulb. Vary how hard you squeeze the bulb, until you get the right amount of suc-

tion: enough to draw the nipple along the pump, but not so much that it is uncomfortable.

6.   Milk should flow out from the nipple pores and collect in the lower part of the pump. Empty the milk often into the sterile container. Do not allow the milk to flow down into the rubber part of the pump.

7.   When little or no additional milk appears, switch to the other breast.

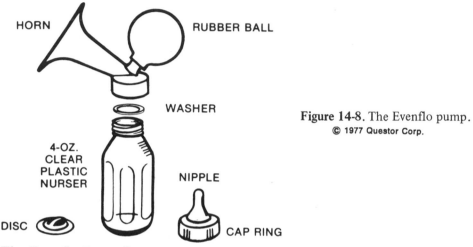

Figure 14-8. The Evenflo pump.
© 1977 Questor Corp.

The Evenflo Breast Pump
The Evenflo breast pump is a modified version of a hand pump. (See Fig. 14-8) It is convenient that the milk goes directly into a small baby-bottle, which attaches to the pump unit. The Evenflo's pump has an additional advantage, the instruction pamphlet "The Joy of Nursing." It may not seem outstanding for a pump to come with instructions, but most pumps come with none at all. The Evenflo pump is used in almost the same way as the standard hand pump.

The Kaneson Expressing and Feeding Bottle
The Kaneson Expressing and Feeding Bottle is an all-plastic, inexpensive device for expressing breast milk (see Fig. 14-9). Included with the unit is a booklet with practical instructions. The two main parts of the unit are plastic cylinders, one of which fits inside the other. The woman holds the unit pressed firmly against her breast with her thumb and forefinger. With the other hand, she moves the ouside cylinder in and out. The piston-type action draws milk from the breast. The inside cylinder may be easily converted to

a feeding bottle by adding the included rubber nipple. Complete instructions for using the unit are included (assembling, sterilizing, etc.).

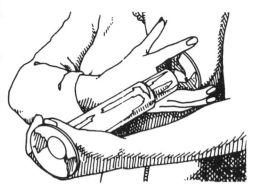

Figure 14-9. The Kaneson Happy pump, from Happy Family Products.

BREAST MASSAGE AND THE HAND-EXPRESSION OF BREAST MILK

The mother wishing to use hand-expression of breast milk should use breast massage to help trigger a let-down and also to help move the milk forward in the breast toward the nipple. If she plans to use the expressed milk for the baby she should have a sterilized container ready.

Instructions for Massage

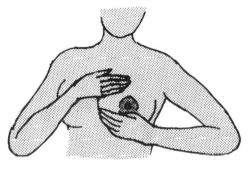

Figure 14-10. Breast massage.

Wash your hands and expose the breasts. Stroke the breast gently but firmly with the palms of the hands. Alternate hands as you work around each breast. Massage from several starting points, always working toward the nipple area. Massage from shoulder down, from under the arm and over, from waist up, and then from center of the chest over to the nipple. Massage around each breast several times.

Some women with large breasts prefer to support the breast with one hand and do breast massage and hand-expression with the other hand.

The time chosen for learning how to hand-express milk can make a big difference. Women who try it right after a nursing, believing that they won't be taking any milk away from the baby, often get discouraged and give up. For the woman who is nursing, the easiest time to learn the skill is *during* a nursing. The let-down has triggered the milk to flow in both breasts and hand-expressing then is psychologically very rewarding. A woman whose baby cannot nurse should be advised to try hand-expression when her breasts have colostrum or milk, but before her breasts become uncomfortably full.

The Hand-Expression of Breast Milk

After having followed the steps of massaging the breasts (above), the woman is ready to hand-express her milk.

Instructions for Hand-Expression of Milk

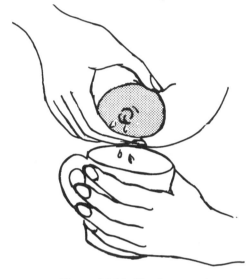

Figure 14-11. Hand-expression.

1. Do breast massage.
2. Place the thumb and index finger on the areola or darker skin around the nipple—about an inch back from the nipple. Press inward toward the chest wall and squeeze the thumb and finger together gently: *push back and squeeze.* Don't slide the thumb and finger. Don't pull the nipple out.
3. Keep the thumb and finger in that position and express until no more drops come out. Then move to another location around the nipple and repeat.
4. Lean over the sterile container and catch the milk. Switch to the other breast and again massage before beginning to express.

Many women have tried to learn hand-expression with little success. There are some common reasons for failure. Many fail to push back toward the chest wall while squeezing. "Push back and squeeze." Many try to learn on empty breasts. Many fail to use massage before hand-expression. Women who have seen a film showing a farmer milking a cow think that they should imitate the way the farmer's hands jerk outward. When they try to milk their breasts in the same way, they fail. A woman may be helped by the correct mental image. It is the baby's mouth *compressing* the sinuses, which lie under the areola, that the woman needs to duplicate.

Women who are engorged in the early days of nursing may want to hand-express to relieve some of the fullness near the nipple. They may find it difficult to learn hand-expression on their firm and tender breasts. The woman should be told to stand in the shower, with her *back* to the water, so that the water runs down over her shoulders. The woman may then be able to hand-express a little. A good substitute for the warm shower can be warm compresses on the breasts, in place of massage, which would be uncomfortable on engorged breasts. Milk flow has also been observed to increase by having the woman immerse her full breast in a pan or sink of warm water or in front of her in a bath. The milk may flow out, whereas it had been only coming out in occasional drops before.

STORING BREAST MILK

The treatment and handling of breast milk varies considerably, depending on whether the milk is handled by only the mother or also by hospital staff who are caring for a premature or ill infant. Donation to milk banks will involve treatment specific to the particular bank. Mothers who collect and store their own milk in order to have it given in a bottle to their own healthy babies would not be following the same procedures as would be required in a hospital setting. In the home, a mother may use equipment that has been washed in hot water, often in a dishwasher, although it is safer for the mother to sterilize the bottles and other collecting jars. If home sterilizing is desired, the woman puts all the clean items into a pan, covers them with cold water, brings the water to a boil, and boils it for five minutes. The water is drained off by using the pan's lid. The inside part of any sterilized container should not be touched.

The milk should be chilled immediately after collection. Milk can be kept in the refrigerator up to 48 hours. If the woman does not plan to use milk in the next day or so, she should place it in the freezer right away.

The freezer ideally should maintain a temperature of 0^0F. If the temperature is 0^0F, the milk can be kept for months.

The usual method for women who are collecting milk for their own baby's use is to collect the milk in different containers each with the right amount for one feeding. A woman with a young baby may save 3½ oz in a 4 oz baby bottle. When she is out, the baby-sitter has the right amount in the bottle. In most cases, women are able to collect only an ounce at one time, although some women can get more. The procedure is to chill the newly expressed milk in its sterilized container in the refrigerator. When it is cold, the new milk is added as a new layer to the already frozen milk in another container. The milk will have a layered look, which is unfamiliar to women who have seen only homogenized cows' milk.

Since the milk needs space in which to expand as it freezes, no container should be filled to the top.

When the milk is to be fed to the baby, it should be taken from the freezer and held under cold, then gradually warmer, water to thaw, while it is being shaken gently. The milk can then be heated to body temperature in a pan of water. The milk should not have been defrosted ahead of time: when the baby starts to stir and the sitter thinks that he is probably hungry, she takes the frozen milk out.

Some women freeze milk in disposable nurser bags. Since these bags were not made for freezing and can split open, the woman must be careful not to overfill each bag.

Collecting and storing milk for a premature or ill infant requires special instructions. The mother may be instructed in the collection of milk at home and be given pre-sterilized containers in which to put the milk. These containers and the parts of the breast pump that come in contact with the milk may be either glass or plastic. The mother should be instructed to bring the milk to the hospital daily since usually the milk is wanted chilled but not frozen. She must be given specific instructions on hand-washing routines,etc.

In other hospitals, mothers of premature infants are asked to come into the hospital to use the electric breast pump, although this arrangement may make it difficult to collect milk at the preferred schedule of every 2-3 hours.

DONOR MILK

There are definite cases where donor breast milk has been life saving to a child with multiple formula intolerance. It has been possible, although difficult, in such cases for the natural mother to relactate and eventually supply her own child's needs. (Relactation is discussed in Chapter 13.)

More often, however, human donor milk is obtained for the pre-term infant. The physician who decides to use human milk in such a case must decide whether to use donor milk or request that the mother supply her own milk. The individual circumstances, the mother's feelings, the advantages of using the mother's own milk shoud be considered in making this decision.

Arguments for the Use of Donor Milk
. . . . for the Premature Infant . . . .

1.   Some mothers find the idea of pumping and/or breast-feeding distasteful.

2.   Some mothers are unable to provide enough milk even shortly after delivery.

3.   Difficulty in maintaining a milk supply over a long period of time is not uncommon, although this difficulty can be prevented or minimized with ideal information on pumping and emotional support.

4.   It is sometimes relatively easy to obtain human milk from a milk bank or from donor mothers.

5.   If the infant has been transported to an intensive care nursery in a hospital some distance from the mother, the

mother's own milk must be taken daily to the hospital at some inconvenience. (In some cases women have had their milk transported, packed in ice, to the hospital by a husband, a neighbor, the baby's grandparent, or other relative, possibly by someone who commuted daily to the city where the hospital is located.)

Why use the mother's own milk?

...... Arguments for Using the Mother's Own Milk.......

1.   Colostrum may be obtained and given to the baby, offering its added immunological protection to the especially immunologically immature premature infant.

2.   There is greater assurance that the milk is free from medications and viruses. Milk may be given fresh, avoiding the need for freezing and/or heat treatment. Living cells and immunoglobulins are left intact.

3.   The mother who is helped to provide her own milk successfully has a psychological advantage; she is likely to find comfort and satisfaction from her unique contribution to her infant's survival (13). Women who have had to depend upon the generosity of donors have been subject to feelings of inadequacy and guilt (17). Even if the baby dies, the bond that was created may help the mother work through the grieving process (13).

More theoretical reasons to favor use of mother's own milk include the concern of graft versus host reaction triggered by living lymphocytes from donor milk in the very immature infant. This may be avoided by destroying the living cells through processing the milk. There are however no documented cases of this reaction to breast milk. Recent observation of a higher nitrogen content in the milk of women delivering prematurely is of note, but at present its significance is unknown. Investigation of protein content of human milk from mothers of premature infants is indicated. Some have claimed that there is a significant decrease in protein content in human milk during the course of lactation, which might be another possible disadvantage to pooled donor milk for the very young infant. Again, further research is indicated.

   Another consideration is the psychological and physical burden placed on the mothers who supply the donor milk and on their families. Those who have actually been involved in this undertaking emphasize the enormous demands of time and attention to sterile procedures necessary in the collection of breast milk.

Clearly, when it is decided to use human milk to feed an individual baby, mother's own milk is optimal. Donor milk is best reserved for cases of true emergency when human milk appears to be life saving and the mother's own milk is not available or safe to use.

MILK BANKS

Milk banks make human milk available to infants who cannot tolerate other foods, to some premature nurseries, and to researchers. The banks receive the milk from donors, who may or may not be paid.

The woman who is donating on a regular basis needs ongoing support; if she becomes discouraged, she is likely to stop pumping. A woman who is both nursing and pumping may require a source of support for both of these different, although related, activities.

The newer special formulas have lessened the need for human milk, so there are fewer banks than in the past. However, the existing banks have many requests for milk and limit the milk they give out to prescriptions. Milk which is contaminated by drugs or bacteria may be given to researchers.

Some hospitals have their own pumps to which mothers are encouraged to go to express their own fresh and unprocessed milk which is used for their own infants (16). The area in the hospital where the pumps and other equipment are located may also be called a milk bank. The majority of banks, however, collect donor milk.

In a 1976 survey of milk banks about their methods of collecting and storing human milk, four different ways of handling donated milk were reported:

. . . . How Milk Banks Handle Human Milk. . . . .

1. using fresh milk, untreated from tested donors

2. using frozen milk, untreated from tested donors

3. using frozen milk, after defrosting, pooling, culturing, and refreezing

4. using frozen milk, after defrosting, pooling, autoclaving and refreezing (17).

At a workshop on the feeding of human milk to premature infants, one of the points of agreement among the participants was that guidelines should be established for the operation of human milk banks (18).

The possibility of bacterial contamination has made heat treatment a common procedure (19). Fort et al concluded that the holder pasteurization process (heating at 62.5°C for 30 minutes) seems to be the method of choice for treating human milk (20). It minimizes the loss of immunoglobulins and other protective proteins, but may inactivate milk lipases (fat absorption is decreased) (21).

Heat treating all human milk may not be necessary. If adequate instructions are given to mothers for collecting and storing "clean milk," heat treating may not be required for milk without bacterial contamination (22).

Any processing of the milk affects some loss of vital elements, with heating destroying both cells and immunoglobulins, and freezing, the cellular elements.

BRA PADS

Some commercial bra pads have a plastic liner, which may be on the outside, or between the layers. This type of bra pad may be good for the woman's dress, but it is harmful to the nipples. Pads that occlude the air are a contributing factor in causing sore nipples and do nothing to help cases of normal newborn soreness. Some women solve the problem (and save the expense of buying pads) by using cotton handkerchiefs.

Reusable cloth bra pads are also available. (See Appendix B) These are two squares of fabric stitched together with an open side for inserting absorbent material, such as paper tissues or handkerchiefs. The fact that these are more economical is secondary. More importantly, they do not occlude the air so they allow sore nipples to heal comfortably. Also, they do not stick to wet nipple/areola skin (wet from leaking), as commercial bra pads do.

LACT-AID

The Lact-Aid Nursing Supplementer was invented to help a woman nurse an adopted baby (see Fig. 14-12). The main problem in trying to nurse an adopted baby, or to relactate, is cajoling the baby to nurse on empty breasts. The Lact-Aid supplies the baby with formula or donated breast milk from a plastic bag supported between the mother's breasts. The milk from the bag is drawn into the baby's mouth through narrow tubing, as he simultaneously suckles at the mother's nipple and at the end of the tubing that lies along side her nipple. Hair-dressing tape may be used to hold the tubing in place if necessary. Because the baby is receiving milk, he obliges the mother by stimulating her breasts to produce milk—unless the infant refuses to nurse even with the Lact-Aid, which may happen with infants who are accustomed to bottles. Relactation is described in Chapter 13.

The written materials that promote the use of the Lact-Aid suggest other uses in addition to nursing adopted babies. For some of these suggestions, however, practical experience has shown mixed or disappointing results. La Leche League, for example, warns against resorting to the use of the Lact-Aid when very frequent nursing would be effective (23). The use of the Lact-Aid could be appropriate to suggest in the following circumstances:

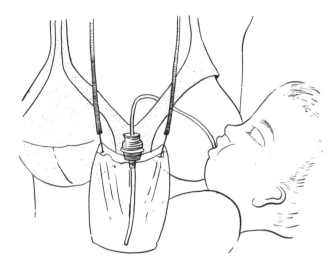

Figure 14-12, The Lact-Aid. Further instructions on use accompany the Lact-Aid.

. . . .Situations when the Lact-Aid might be Appropriate . . . .

1.   An adoptive mother who wants to initiate breastfeeding.

2.   A mother who wants to initiate breastfeeding although her baby has been on a bottle.

3.   A mother who has stopped breastfeeding for a period of time and wants to return to it (23).

4.   A mother whose nursing baby is failing to thrive because of inadequate milk supply (24).

References

1.   Newton, N: *The Family Book of Child Care*. New York: Harper & Row, 1957.

2.   Haire, D: The Nurse's Contribution to Successful Breast-Feeding and the Medical Value of Breast-Feeding. Chapter V of *Implementing Family Centered Maternity Care*, International Childbirth Education Association, 1974.

3. Applebaum, RM: Breast Feeding and Care of the Breasts. Reprinted from Davis' *Gynecology and Obstetrics,* Vol. I, Chapter 32, Hagerstown, Maryland: Harper & Row, Inc., 1974.

4. Newton, M and Newton, N: The Normal Course and Management of Lactation, Clin. Obstet. Gynecol. 5 (1): March, 1962.

5. Applebaum, RM: The physician and a common sense approach to breast feeding, South. Med. J. 63:793, 1970.

6. Worrell, M: Pacifiers. Leaven, Franklin Park, IL: La Leche League International, July-August, 1975.

7. Abler, M: About Pacifiers. Leaven, Franklin Park, IL: La Leche League International, May-June, 1972.

8. Wolff, P: Sucking patterns of infant mammals, Brain Behav. Evol. 1:354, 1968.

9. Countryman, BA: How the Maternity Nurse Can Help the Breastfeeding Mother. Franklin Park, IL: La Leche League International, 1977.

10. Waller, H: The Early Failure of Breastfeeding: A clinical Study of its causes and their prevention, Arch. Dis. Child. 21:1, 1946.

11. Choi, MV: Breast milk for infants who can't breastfeed, Am. J. Nurs. 78:852, 1978.

12. Newton, M and Egli, GE: The effect of intranasal administration of oxytocin on the letdown of milk in lactating women, Am. J. Obstet. Gynecol. 76:103, 1958.

13. Auerbach, K, coordinator: Breastfeeding the premature infant, Keeping Abreast Journal II (2) April-June, 1977.

14. Pitt, J: Breast milk leucocytes, Pediatr. 58: 769, 1976.

15. Liebhaber, M et al: Comparison of bacterial contamination with two methods of human milk collection, J. Pediatr. 92:236, 1978.

16. Fleischaker, JW et al: The Louisville breast milk program, Keeping Abreast Journal II (2): 124, April-June, 1977.

17. Popper, B and Countryman, BA: Establishing an institutional milk bank. Franklin Park, IL: La Leche League International, 1977.

18. Panelists: Human milk in premature infant feeding: summary of a workshop, Pediatr. 57: 741, 1976.

19. Leading article: Heating human milk, Br. Med. J. 1:1372, 1977.

20. Ford, JE et al: Influence of the heat treatment of human milk on some of its protective constituents, J.Pediatr. 90:29, 1977.

21. Williamson, S et al: Effect of heat treatment of human milk on absorption of nitrogen, fat, sodium, and calcium, phosphorus by pre term infants, Arch. Dis. Child. 53:555, 1978.

22. Ikonen, RS and Maki, K: (Letter in response to heating human milk), Br. Med. J. 2:386, 1977.

23. Use of the Lact-Aid Supplementer, Franklin Park, IL: La Leche League International, 1977.

24. Weichert, CE: Lactational Reflex Recovery in breastfeeding failure, Pediatr. 63 (5):799, 1979.

APPENDIX A

RESOURCES FOR PROFESSIONALS AND MOTHERS

Recommended Additional Reading for the Professional

1. Cowie, AT and Tindal, JS: *The Physiology of Lactation.* Baltimore: Williams & Wilkins, 1971.

2. CIBA Foundation Symposium no. 45 (new series). *Breast-Feeding and the Mother.* Amsterdam: Elsevier, 1976.

3. Dunn, J: *Distress and Comfort.* Cambridge, MA: Harvard University Press, 1977.

4. Haire, D: The Nurse's Contribution to Successful Breast-Feeding and The Medical Value of Breast-Feeding in *Implementing Family Centered Maternity Care.* ICEA, 1974.

5. Jelliffe, DB and Jelliffe, P: *Human Milk in the Modern World.* London: Oxford Press, 1978.

6. Josimovich, J et al: *Lactogenic Hormones, Fetal Nutrition and Lactation.* New York: John Wiley and Sons, 1974.

7. Klaus, MH and Kennell, J: *Maternal-Infant Bonding.* Saint Louis: The C.V. Mosby Company, 1976.

8. Kon, SK and Cowie, AT: *Milk: The Mammary Gland and Its Secretion* (Vols. I and II). New York: Academic Press, 1961.

9. Parkes, AS et al: (eds.) Fertility Regulation during Human Lactation. Journal of Biosocial Science Supplement No. 4. P.O. Box 32, Commerce Way, Colchester CO2 8PH, England.

10. Pediatric Clinics of North America, Vol. 24, No. 1. Symposium on Nutrition in Pediatrics, Feb., 1977.

11. Vorherr, H: *The Breast.* New York: Academic Press, 1974.

Books on Breastfeeding Recommended for Mothers

1. Brewster, DP: *You Can Breastfeed Your Baby...Even in Special Situations.* Emmaus, PA: Rodale Press, 1979.

2. Eiger, MS and Olds, Sally: *The Complete Book of Breastfeeding*. New York: Workman Publishing Co., Inc., 1972.

3. La Leche League International: The Womanly Art of Breastfeeding. Franklin Park, Illinois: LLL, 1963.

4. Pryor, K: *Nursing Your Baby*. New York: Pocket Book Division of Simon & Schuster, 1973.

5. Phillips, V. *Successful Breast Feeding*. Victoria, Australia: Nursing Mothers' Association of Australia, 1976.

6. Raphael, D: *The Tender Gift: Breastfeeding*. Englewood Cliffs, New Jersey: Prentice Hall, 1973.

Sources of Inexpensive Pamphlets as Teaching Aids on Breastfeeding

1. Health Education Associates
   520 School House Lane
   Willow Grove, PA 19090 USA

2. ICEA Bookcenter
   P.O. Box 70258
   Seattle, WA 98107 USA

3. La Leche League International
   9616 Minneapolis Avenue
   Franklin Park, IL 60131 USA

4. Nursing Mothers Association of Australia
   P.O. Box 230
   Hawthorne, Victoria 3122
   Australia

APPENDIX B

RESOURCES FOR DEVICES AND OTHER PRODUCTS

Breast Pumps

1. Egnell, Inc.
   412 Park Avenue
   Cary, IL 60013 USA
   (Egnell has local rental
   depots and will supply
   a list.)

   Rental Distributor in England:
   The National Childbirth Trust
   9, Queensborough Terrace
   Bayswater
   London W2 3TB

   Sales Distributor in England
   Eschmann Bros & Walsh Limited
   Peter Rd.
   Lancing, Sussex BN15 8TJ

2. Other electric breast pumps
   can be rented from medical
   supply houses (Yellow Pages).

3. Loyd-B Pump:
   Lopuco, Ltd.
   1615 Old Annapolis Road
   Woodbine, MD 21797 USA

4. Small hand pumps are available at
   pharmacies.

5. Evenflo breast pump:
   Some pharmacies, through Sears
   stores, and the Sears catalogue.

6. Kaneson Expressing and Feeding Bottle:
   Happy Family Products
   1252 S. La Cienega Blvd.
   Los Angeles, CA 90035 USA

   Yanase Waitch K.K.
   9-12, Higashitenma 1 chome
   Kita-ku, Osaka 530
   Japan

Marshall Electronics, Inc.
Clayton Division
7440 North Long Avenue
Skokie, IL 60076 USA

Kimal Scientific Products Ltd.
Kimal House
Uxbridge Road
Hillingdon Health
Middlesex UB10 OPW
England

Milk Cup (Woolwich Shield in England)

CEA of Greater Philadelphia
129 Fayette Street
Conshohocken, PA 19428 USA

La Leche League International
9616 Minneapolis Avenue
Franklin Park, IL 60131 USA
(available by the term "breast
shield")

Reusable Bra Pads

CEA of Greater Philadelphia
129 Fayette Street
Conshohocken, PA 19428 USA

Lact-Aid

Lact-Aid is available only through the
mail.
    Lact-Aid
    Box 6861
    Denver, CO 80206 USA

Other Products (available through
            pharmacies)

1. The Nuk Exercisor (pacifier) and
    Nuk bottle nipples.

2. Disposable bra pads

3. Nipple shields, breast shields

4. The Natural Nursing Nipple Shield
    is used in England.

APPENDIX C

ADDRESSES OF BREASTFEEDING SUPPORT ORGANIZATIONS

Ammehjelpen
Postboks 15
Holmen, Oslo 3, Norway
(Support group for breastfeeding
mothers)

Caring
P.O. Box 400
Milton, WI 98354 USA
(Help for parents of children with
Down's Syndrome)

C/SEC, Inc.
23 Cedar Street
Cambridge, MA 02140 USA
(Support group for mothers who
deliver by cesarean section)

Health Education Associates
520 School House Lane
Willow Grove, PA 19090 USA
(Continuing education programs on
breastfeeding management for hospital staff members)

Human Lactation Center Ltd.
666 Sturges Highway
Westport, CT 06880 USA
(Special interest in breastfeeding
in Third World countries

International Childbirth Education
Association (ICEA)
P.O. Box 10852
Milwaukee, WI 53220 USA
(Affiliated, separate childbirth groups,
many offering breastfeeding support)

ICEA Book Center
P.O. Box 70258
Seattle, WA 98107 USA
(Large selection of books on breastfeeding, childbirth, parenting mail-
order book list, news and reviews free
with self-addressed, stamped envelope)

La Leche League International
9616 Minneapolis Avenue
Franklin Park, IL 50131 USA
(Largest breastfeeding support group,
with thousands of local groups)

National Organization of Mothers of
Twins Clubs, Inc.
3402 Amberwood Lane
Rockville, MD 20853 USA
(Clubs for mothers of twins)

National Childbirth Trust
Breast-feeding Promotion Group
9 Queensborough Terrace
London W2 3TB, England
(Lay group for childbirth and breast-
feeding support)

National Foundation-March of Dimes
P.O. Box 2000
White Plains, NY 10602 USA
(Has materials on nutrition, preg-
nancy, etc.)

Nursing Mothers' Association of
of Australia
P.O. Box 230
Hawthorn, Victoria 3122, Australia
(A breastfeeding support group for
mothers)

Index

* * * * * * * * * * * * * *